"I'm Pregnant, Now What Do I Do?"

Foreword by Elizabeth C. Winship, author of
the nationally syndicated column for teens, **"Ask Beth"**

"I'm Pregnant, Now What Do I Do?"

ROBERT W. BUCKINGHAM, DR. P.H.
& MARY P. DERBY, R.N., M.P.H.

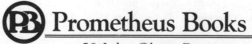 **Prometheus Books**
59 John Glenn Drive
Amherst, New York 14228-2197

Cover photos courtesy of the following organizations:

National Adoption Information Clearinghouse, 5640 Nicholson Lane, Suite 300, Rockville, MD 20852 (photo of adoptive family)

Expressions Studio of Photography, 1277 Hertel Avenue, Buffalo, NY 14216 (photo of couple)

March of Dimes Birth Defects Foundation, 1275 Mamaroneck Avenue, White Plains, NY 10605 (all other photos)

Published 1997 by Prometheus Books

01 00 99 98 97   5 4 3 2 1

Library of Congress Cataloging-in-Publication Data

Buckingham, Robert W.
    "I'm pregnant, now what do I do?" / by Robert W. Buckingham and Mary P. Derby.
        p.   cm.
    Summary: Discusses the feelings and circumstances of and possible options for
teenagers who become pregnant and describes the experiences of young women who kept
their babies, who had abortions, and who gave their babies up for adoption.
    ISBN 1–57392–117–3 (pbk. : alk. paper)
    1. Teenage mothers—United States—Juvenile literature. 2. Teenage mothers—
United States—Case studies—Juvenile literature. 3. Teenage pregnancy—Psychological
aspects—Juvenile literature. 4. Abortion—Psychological aspects—Juvenile literature.
5. Adoption—Psychological aspects—Juvenile literature. [1. Pregnancy. 2. Teenage
mothers. 3. Adoption. 4. Abortion.] I. Derby, Mary P. II. Title.
HQ759.4.B83   1996
306.874'3—dc21   96–48344
                                                                         CIP
                                                                          AC

Printed in the United States of America on acid-free paper

This book is dedicated to
all those young women
who face the choice.

Contents

Acknowledgments — 9

Foreword — 11

1. What Now? — 15

2. Just the Facts — 36

3. Deciding What's Right for Me — 64

4. Becoming a Parent — 84

5. Is Abortion the Right Choice for Me? — 105

6. Considering Adoption? — 127

7. Case Studies: Raising a Child — 145

8. Case Studies: Choosing Abortion — 158

9. Case Studies: Placing a Child for Adoption — 172

10. Your Partner's Responsibility — 186

11. Moving Forward — 204

Glossary — 213

Resources — 221

Acknowledgments

We would like to acknowledge the many people who through their contributions helped make this book possible and rewarding for those who may read it. First, our deepest appreciation is extended to the individuals who shared their personal experiences. It is their stories and their lives which give this book its real meaning and value.

Second, we would like to recognize the invaluable input of two very special women, Susan Desilet and Lora Oakes Chatfield, CNM, MPH. They are both truly talented and remarkable women whose insight, support, and encouragement, along with their wisdom and humor helped to keep this book moving forward.

Many others gave generously of their time in providing assistance in their area of expertise, and their contribution is sincerely appreciated: Caroline Stone, DNSc, RN c.; Lisa Gurland, RN, PsyD; and Abigail English, JD, at the National Center for Youth Law. A special thank you to others who provided invaluable comments and encouragement: Martha Magner, RN; Sterling Anderson, MEd; Laura Grayzel, RN; and Elsa Marcus. Many thanks to Jennifer Coate of the March of Dimes, Debra G. Smith of the National Adoption Information Clearinghouse, and Melissa Pouridas of the American College of Obstetricians and Gynecologists for providing us with the respective photographs/illustrations from their agencies.

And, last but not least, we would like to thank a team of truly dedicated professionals at Prometheus Books, Kathy McGuinness-Deyell for her hard work and dedication, Steven Mitchell for his commitment to excellence, and Dan Wasinger for his constant inspiration.

Foreword

Although there are quite a few books for teenagers about what happens when you get pregnant, there are many good reasons to pick this one. It's up-to-date. It has all the facts. And most important, it is written about real girls who faced this all-too-real situation. Reading about their experiences, their ideas, and their choices is the best way for a young woman to find out what the right decision for someone in this situation is.

In the last few years there has been a revolutionary change in the amount of knowledge about human sexuality available to young people. Sex education is now taught in many more schools. There is more public information about contraception. It may seem that we couldn't possibly need yet another book on teenage pregnancy, but we sure do! We in the United States still have the highest rate of adolescent pregnancy in the developed world. Many mothers, and most fathers, still find it difficult to really talk to their children about sex. While there has been much improvement in sex education in our schools, it isn't always very complete or, alas, very forthcoming. Insufficient knowledge about sex is coupled today with huge pressure in the media to be sexy. So long as we tolerate runaway sexiness in the media, we give kids the message that sex is something everyone does, so why shouldn't they do it too? The result? Every year about one million teenaged girls unintentionally become pregnant.

One reason for this is that desire runs way ahead of common sense. Another is that adolescents find it very hard to believe that anything bad could ever happen to them. This so-called magical thinking makes it all the more necessary for young people to learn "The Facts." Many of them just don't understand the importance of either waiting for sex or using effective contraception.

Much of the literature in print and the lessons about sex for these young people somehow misses the mark. This book, with its simply expressed, yet thorough explanations about sex, and its frequent referral to the actual experiences of adolescents, is an exception. It will be of great help to girls and boys contemplating having sex and it also has the necessary information for teens who are already involved sexually and those girls who are pregnant and wondering what to do about it.

Accidental pregnancy still occurs to over a million teenage girls a year in our country. Three million teenagers become infected with a sexually transmitted disease each year. Instead of emphasizing shame and fear as a reaction to these events, the authors urge girls to develop a positive attitude. Except for the occasional miscarriage, pregnancies don't just go away by themselves. It is necessary for girls to cope. Dr. Buckingham and Ms. Derby urge girls to embrace this opportunity to make a big decision, one which will change their lives.

Many young pregnant girls are so panicked they can't think straight. The authors tell them how to find somebody who can present a realistic picture of what it's like to raise a child. The pregnant teen needs experienced, practical, and understanding help in deciding among her three choices: adoption, abortion, or raising her child herself. A teenaged father is not always able or even willing to help. He's not pregnant!

There is real help here about how to make this tremendous decision which should help conquer the terrible fear that most pregnant teenagers feel. This fear often immobilizes girls so they don't get help, and don't make any decisions when there is still time to include abortion as one opportunity. Is abortion always the right answer? It certainly is an important available option, but in some cases adoption would be better. Raising the child at home may be appealing, but is extremely demanding on a young mother. There is no preference given here for any one of these three choices. Instead, the authors describe realistically and frankly what each choice entails.

The book includes case studies of several girls who tried different ways of coping with their pregnancy, and how they fared. This is the best way for a teenager to learn how her future life will be affected under different circumstances. If you are considering an abortion, put yourself in the same shoes as Courtney. Read why she made this choice, and how she felt about it. If you think adoption is the answer, finding out how it went for Carolyn will give you food for thought. And if you feel you should raise a child yourself, read about Jennifer and how she handled being a hands-on mother. There are other case studies of girls who tried the different options. There is also information about family and friends and the boyfriends who fathered the children.

Most important, perhaps, this whole book provides excellent information to teens who are considering having sexual intercourse. So many young people do not take the risks into account. If a teen reads *"I'm Pregnant, Now What Do I Do?"* it will be impossible for him or her not to understand the consequences.

—Elizabeth C. Winship,
Author of the nationally syndicated column "Ask Beth"

1

What Now?

... it used to be that getting pregnant when you weren't married ruined your life because of the disgrace, now ...[1]

Sara sat alone in her bedroom crying. Her period was almost two months late. Each morning for the past several days she had felt nauseated, and at times she had been sick to her stomach. Her breasts ached. The home pregnancy test she had taken that morning was positive. Sara was in shock, and wondered how this could have happened to her, at her age. She thought back to the one time she had had sex with her boyfriend, Andy. It had been his first time too. How did she get pregnant the first time she'd had sex? No one could possibly be so unlucky, she thought. She was sure the pregnancy test must be wrong, but then she remembered that they hadn't used birth control. It had been the end of the summer. Andy was leaving for college. They were celebrating. They were both nervous, and got caught up in the moment. She didn't want to bring up birth control. They were having a special time. She didn't want to ruin it. Besides she had wanted to show him that she was mature, and just as grown-up as the college women she knew he would be meeting soon. Now I'm pregnant, sobbed Sara. How could I have let this happen? How could I have been so stupid? What am I supposed to do now? My life is ruined.

Sara didn't know who to turn to. Normally she would turn to her mom when she needed help; they had a good relationship. She struggled with whether she should turn to her mom now. She felt ashamed and guilty, and

15

she worried about telling her mom. Her mother was going through a divorce, and the last thing Sara wanted to do was burden her mom with her pregnancy. She didn't want to add to the stress. Sara was afraid that the news of her pregnancy would destroy her mother. Sara thought about talking to one of her friends. Who could she trust? Her boyfriend Andy was a freshman in college. She was a sophomore in high school. Her friends didn't like Andy; they thought he was too old for her. She wasn't sure how he would react. She was afraid their relationship would end, and then what would she do? She wondered if Andy would want to be a father now, or would he abandon her?

Sara is not alone. Lots of teens become pregnant the first time they have sex because they do not use birth control. About 20 percent of all teens who become pregnant do so within one month of the first time they had sexual intercourse. Many of these teens react just like Sara did. They are angry, confused, and in shock. They are overwhelmed with their feelings. They're not sure whom they should talk to or whom they can trust.

In chapter 7, you will read about Jennifer, who shared her experience. She was seventeen and a senior in high school when she got pregnant. She was older than Sara, but she felt the same feelings of shame, guilt, and fear. She was afraid to tell her parents and felt that she had disappointed them. This is what Jennifer had to say:

I got pregnant the very first time I had sex, so I really felt unlucky. I felt like the odds were against me. I felt stupid and ashamed because I knew about contraceptives. I remember feeling awkward about my body. I hadn't planned to have sex so I wasn't prepared. My boyfriend and I had never talked about birth control. I didn't know how to tell my boyfriend to use a condom. . . . I was afraid to tell my parents. I knew they were going to be really upset. I knew I had disappointed them. I knew they would be afraid for me and the fate of my child.

Other teens become pregnant because they don't know how a pregnancy happens. There are a lot of misconceptions among teens about how to prevent a pregnancy. Some teens mistakenly believe that you can't get pregnant if you have sex standing up, if you have sex when you're very young or haven't gotten your period yet, or if you douche after you have sex. Some are willing to trust their boyfriend that he will withdraw or "pull out" on time. Jill says: "That's what I did. He told me, 'Don't worry, honey, it will be perfectly all right.' Well it wasn't. I got pregnant that night." Others take risks and think they will be okay because they're certain that they've calculated their "safe days," and think they are avoiding sex on days they believe they are fertile. This is an unreliable method. If this happened to you, there's no reason to feel stupid. Other teens have similar misconceptions and become pregnant when they don't want to.

Still other teens don't use contraception because they mistakenly believe they don't need to. They were lucky and didn't get pregnant the first time, so they took more chances, thinking that "it couldn't happen to them." This happened to Alison, who was fourteen years old when she became pregnant. She shares her experience in chapter 8. Here's what Alison had to say:

> I knew all about birth control. I knew other kids in my class who had dropped out of school because they were pregnant. I just didn't bother to take any precautions. I figured I was too young to get pregnant. I wasn't like the "other girls" in my class who were always getting themselves into trouble. . . . I didn't get pregnant right away. That's another reason why I took so many chances. I really thought it couldn't happen to me. So each and every time we had sex I was willing to take a chance. . . . We had sex quite a few times before I actually got pregnant.

Alison is not alone. About 50 percent of all teens who become pregnant for the first time become pregnant within six months of their first sexual experience. Many teens feel pressure to have sex. They think all their friends are sexually active, or they want to experiment and find out what it's all about. Unfortunately many begin sexual activity not fully understanding the responsibility and consequences of such activity. Many are shocked when they find they are pregnant when they didn't intend to become pregnant. They are faced with making a very difficult decision at a time in their lives when they don't feel prepared to.

There are other teens who do use birth control, at least some of the time. According to the Alan Guttmacher Institute,* two-thirds of teens use some form of birth control, usually the male condom, the first time they have sexual intercourse.[2] Sometimes teens make an attempt to use birth control, but they don't use it consistently and correctly every time they have sexual intercourse. Many teens don't anticipate having sex, so they don't prepare themselves. Many teens, like Cheryl, mistakenly believe that if you prepare yourself it's less romantic and less spontaneous. Cheryl says:

---

*The Alan Guttmacher Institute is a not-for-profit corporation for reproductive health research and public education.

It's a hard thing to talk about. You don't want to spoil the moment. I know it's not right, but sometimes you can get careless, and not take precautions. If you've been in a relationship for a few months, and for whatever reason you stopped taking precautions, you don't feel comfortable bringing up the issue again, you worry about what your boyfriend is thinking. You're wondering if he thinks you don't trust him, or you wonder if he won't trust you, if he thinks you're seeing someone else.

When these teens do become pregnant, they are as shocked and disappointed with themselves as young women are who don't use birth control. They feel very bad about getting pregnant and are hard on themselves. Carolyn shares her experience in chapter 9. She became pregnant at age sixteen. She had been taking the pill for about a year, but Carolyn said:

> I kept forgetting to take my pills. I knew I was supposed to use back-up protection, but I didn't bother. I was preoccupied with our relationship. My boyfriend, Dave, had just received a football scholarship from a college on the West Coast. I knew it would be hard for us to get together and I was worried that our relationship wouldn't last. . . . I cried and cried when the nurse told me I was pregnant. I couldn't believe that I had let this happen. I had been on the pill for about a year, and until I was preoccupied about Dave leaving, I was always responsible about taking it. I felt good about that. But when I found out I was pregnant, I was devastated. I thought I had been so stupid to have forgotten to take my pills. I could have prevented the pregnancy. I blamed myself. I should have known better.

Some young women wanted to become pregnant. Sometimes a young woman makes the conscious choice to become pregnant, and sometimes it's an unconscious choice. Some teens want a baby so that they will have "someone to love" (and someone to love them); other teens want to begin motherhood at an early age. Maria says, "I'm seventeen. I just got pregnant. I'll be graduating from high school in a few months. My boyfriend will be too. We're planning on getting married. I'm ready to be a mother. This is what I planned."

Other teens want to prove their independence to their parents, but having a baby at a young age doesn't give you independence, it increases your dependence. It increases your dependence on an adult because you don't yet have all the resources you need to raise a child. Other teens are angry at their parents, and use sex as a way of getting revenge. Wendy says, "My parents are so uptight. They're always trying to control what I do. I hate it. It was almost worth getting pregnant, just to see the expressions on their faces."

The vast majority of teens who become pregnant say they did not intend to. Almost all teens feel devastated about their pregnancies, and many young women describe feeling numb, in shock, and having difficulty believing what has happened to them. They describe emotions such as feeling ashamed, guilty, stupid, and sad. They feel alone. These feelings are all normal. Becoming pregnant at a young age when you didn't intend to is a very scary thing to happen. If you're like the other young women who have shared their experiences, it's likely that you're feeling bad about yourself and about your pregnancy. You may wish you had done something differently. You may feel ashamed. You may be worried about telling your parents, your guardian, and/or your boyfriend. You may be feeling anxious, not sure how they will react. You may fear that your life is forever ruined, that your life has now changed in a way that you're not so sure you will like.

You may find these emotions overwhelming. It may be hard for you to feel good about yourself right now. These feelings are all normal. There's a lot to think about now. There are a lot of decisions to make. A lot of young women don't feel good about themselves when this happens to them, but *you are a good person. Your life is not ruined. It's taken an unexpected twist or turn, but your life is certainly not over. Your life will be changed in some way no matter what you decide to do, but your life is not over.*

Sometimes an experience like an unintended pregnancy happens in our lives and causes us pain. At these times we can be very hard on ourselves. It's common to feel bad about ourselves, to feel we let ourselves down, to feel we let our parents down, or we let someone else close to us down. We wonder why we didn't do something differently. We second-guess ourselves. We're filled with self-doubts. Suddenly we don't feel capable of doing anything right. This can happen whenever we experience anything unexpectedly, such as an unintended pregnancy. Sometimes we feel our situation is worse because it seems like everything is going wrong all at the same time. For instance, you're fighting with your parents, you fail an important test in school, you come in second in a track meet, you break up with your boyfriend, you have a fight with your best friend, there is a death in your family, or your parents split up. These are stressful experiences. When they happen at the same time you're faced with an unintended pregnancy, it makes each experience seem even more overwhelming. Many teens worry that their life is doomed. This experience will change your life. You will hurt. You will experience a loss and feel pain. You will grieve for a while. And it's normal to have these feelings. It's part of life. All these experiences shape us; they are opportunities. We can learn from these opportunities. We can grow from them. We can change from them and we can become better people. Or, we can choose to feel hurt and defeated by our experiences. There is always a choice. You can work very hard to improve your situation for the best possible outcome, or you can give up and accept whatever comes your way. The choice is always yours. *You are capable of determining what is best for you. You can make a good decision.*

When you first discover that you are pregnant, you may want to cry and shelter yourself for a while like Sara did. It's okay to have a good cry. It may make you feel better. It's okay to be by yourself for a while, to think about and absorb everything that has happened to you. Becoming pregnant at a young age is a crisis for many women. When a crisis happens in our lives, there are typical ways we respond and react. Some of these responses are shock, denial, anger, and guilt. *Realize that you can cope, and that you will do okay.*

The first response typically felt is shock. All the young women who described their experiences spoke about being in shock. Your body feels numb. You're having difficulty absorbing what has happened. Like Sara, you may want to be by yourself for a while. You may find it difficult to talk to anyone else about what has happened. You may not have friends you think you can trust. Like Sara, you may be experiencing some difficulty at home and not want to talk to your parents. Courtney shares her experience in chapter 8. This is how she felt:

> I felt miserable. . . . I felt alone, afraid, and overwhelmed. I was probably in shock. I was on automatic pilot. My actions were robotlike. I went to work and went to classes. I did everything that I would normally do. . . . I was a very private person. . . . I found it tremendously difficult to discuss my situation with anyone other than Steve [the baby's father]. Don't get me wrong, Steve and I were not emotionally intimate, then or ever. We never had a meaningful or mature discussion about the pregnancy or our feelings for each other. However, there was no one else I could turn to. I wasn't close to my family, so I didn't feel I could turn to my parents or any of my brothers and sisters for support. I was also hesitant to turn to my friends.

When something bad happens to us, we often think we can't share our experiences with others, that somehow we did something so wrong that no one else will accept us. Yet at some point in our lives, we will all experience a crisis. Everyone does. We all need people, and when we are experiencing something traumatic in our lives we need people the most.

The next response many young women have is denial. You may experience this. You may be having a hard time comprehending intellectually what has happened to you. Sara described how she felt after she found out she was pregnant. She knew the pregnancy test she took was positive, yet she still had trouble believing that she was really pregnant. A little denial at first is normal. It's a defense mechanism. It cushions and protects you from the shock of your experience. It may help you to regroup and get some of your strength and energy back so you can begin your decision-making process. Some young women stay in denial throughout the entire pregnancy. This, of course, is not normal, and it's not good for you. If you plan on continuing your pregnancy, it can have negative consequences for both you and your baby. Every day you spend in denial you limit the choices that you have.

You do have choices. You can decide what you want to do. You can continue your pregnancy and either raise your baby or place him for adoption; or you can choose to terminate your pregnancy. There are time limits with these choices of which you need to be aware. There is a point in your pregnancy when you can no longer exercise your right to terminate your pregnancy. If you deny that you're pregnant you are limiting the choices that you will be able to make.

There are a lot of reasons why some young women deny their pregnancy. Sometimes they don't recognize pregnancy symptoms and so they don't realize that they are pregnant. Sometimes they are so fearful of how their families will respond to their pregnancies that they hide their pregnancies. With each passing day that they are able to hide their pregnancy, they begin to really believe that they are not pregnant. This can last a short time, or it can last the entire pregnancy. This is not a healthy way to respond to your pregnancy for you or for your baby.

Theresa became pregnant at age fourteen and didn't realize she was pregnant until she went into labor. It was a frightening experience for her. She says:

> I never realized I was pregnant. I remember having sex once with this guy. It was a stupid thing to do, so I blocked the entire experience out of my mind. My periods were always irregular. I was glad I had stopped getting them. I thought I had just gained some more weight. I was always on the heavy side. I never suspected I was pregnant. One night I started having really bad cramps. My mother brought me to the emergency room. After examining me, they knew I was pregnant. I delivered my baby about ten hours later. Everything happened so fast. It was so scary. I didn't have time

to think about what was happening to me. I didn't have time to prepare myself. All of a sudden I was fourteen, and I had a baby to care for.

Some young women, like Theresa, do not realize they are pregnant because they do not recognize common pregnancy symptoms. *The first sign that a woman is pregnant is usually one or more missed menstrual periods. Other common pregnancy symptoms which a young woman may experience include nausea with or without vomiting; swollen, tender breasts; urinating more often than usual; and feeling more tired than usual.* If you suspect for any reason that you might be pregnant, it's best for you to have a pregnancy test done right away. *You may not experience all of these symptoms when you are pregnant.* You can have a pregnancy test done in any family planning clinic, such as Planned Parenthood; a neighborhood health center; an adolescent clinic at your local hospital; or by your regular health care provider. You can read in more detail about pregnancy tests in chapter 2.

Jeannica hid her pregnancy from her mother until she was six months pregnant. Jeannica knew her mother had high expectations for her and she was afraid her mother would not want her to raise her baby. Jeannica said:

I hid my pregnancy from my mom. I know people say you can't do that. I laugh when I hear that because I know you can. That's what I did. I wore big, baggy clothes. I avoided her as much as possible. I wouldn't face her, so she never had the chance to see how big my belly was getting. She finally found out when I was six months pregnant. She walked into my room while I was changing. I was relieved once it was finally out in the open—it was a hassle hiding my pregnancy. I was exhausted from it. My mom brought me right away to the doctor. I didn't realize how much she really cared about me. She wanted what was best for me and my baby.

These young women were lucky. They did not experience any serious complications. They are healthy and their babies are healthy. All young women are not as fortunate as they were. Veronica suspected she was pregnant. She had been pregnant once before, so she knew what to expect. This was not a planned pregnancy, and she ignored her symptoms. She didn't get a pregnancy test. She didn't seek medical attention right away when she didn't feel well. She had an ectopic (tubal) pregnancy.* She had a serious medical complication from her pregnancy which required surgery. Veronica explains:

---

*This type of pregnancy, which is abnormal and can have serious medical consequences, is discussed in more detail in chapter 2.

I suspected I was pregnant right away when I didn't get my period on time. I didn't want to be pregnant. I had gotten pregnant the year before and had had an abortion. I was upset with myself for letting the same thing happen again. Even when I started getting sick in the morning I denied my pregnancy. I started bleeding, but it wasn't like a normal period. I was also having some abdominal pain. For some reason I ignored how I was feeling. I remember being happy, thinking I finally had my period, and that I had worried for nothing. The abdominal pain got worse. I couldn't ignore it anymore. By the time I saw a doctor I was very ill. I had to go to the hospital right away. I had a tubal pregnancy. My tube ruptured. I needed surgery. I lost my tube. Now it will be harder for me to get pregnant when I'm ready to have a baby.

If you suspect you are pregnant, get a pregnancy test right away. If you aren't pregnant, you will be relieved, and you can stop worrying needlessly. If you are pregnant you can get counseling and start thinking about what you want to do. *An early pregnancy diagnosis has its advantages:* you will have more options available to you; you can decrease the chances of serious complications occurring in your pregnancy; you can start taking good care of yourself right away which will benefit both you and your baby; or, you can choose to terminate your pregnancy.

Anger is another common response which many young women feel. Many young women wonder "Why me, why now? Why is this happening?" Anger is a normal and healthy response. You may be angry with yourself, and wish you had taken more precautions. You may be angry with your boyfriend. Perhaps you feel he should have been more responsible, or perhaps he wants you to choose an option which goes against what you want to do. You may also be angry because right now you are forced to make a decision. Your pregnancy will not go away on its own. You will have to make a decision, and no one can make it for you. Whenever we make a decision, we are faced with uncertainties. We never know for sure whether we will be happy with whatever we choose to do. We may feel a loss of control, and that makes us angry.

Monica shares her experience in chapter 9. She became pregnant with her second child when she was twenty. Monica was experiencing other difficulties in her life at the time. She voluntarily gave custody of her first child to her parents so the child could be well cared for while Monica tended to her own needs. Monica was not happy about her second pregnancy, and was angry at herself for getting pregnant. She explains:

> I was very disappointed in myself for getting pregnant. I felt stupid, like I should have known better. I was supposed to be getting my life together, and instead I got pregnant. I was very angry with myself. I kept thinking, why now? Why did I let this happen? I should have known better. I was distraught. I felt very vulnerable. My emotions were all over the place.

Don't let your anger control you. Realize that anger is normal. Find healthy ways to express it. Talk about how you're feeling with someone you trust. Do something special for yourself.

Almost all the young women who shared their experiences felt some form of guilt about their pregnancy. Many felt they had done something wrong. Many felt they had hurt and disappointed their families, and felt bad about that. Sherrie felt particularly guilty about her pregnancy. She found out that she was pregnant at the end of her senior year in high school. She had plans to go away to college. Her mother and her father both worked two jobs to be able to send her to college. They didn't have college degrees, but they wanted their daughter to have a chance in life that they didn't have. Sherrie explains:

> I was quite sad for some time. I was depressed and felt very bad about my pregnancy. Both of my parents had two jobs. They worked very hard and were saving all their money so that I could go to college. They never had that chance. They wanted so much for me to succeed. For years they had willingly made sacrifices, knowing that I would have an opportunity for a better life. I felt very guilty about my pregnancy. I felt I had let my parents down and they had such high expectations for me.

If you feel guilty that you've let someone down, let them know. If you feel comfortable with that person, tell them directly, if not, write them a letter. Realize that guilty feelings are normal. Accept them. Accept yourself. In time your feelings will pass.

Feelings of sadness, shock, anger, and guilt are all normal and can cause you to feel scared and overwhelmed. Every woman who is pregnant is afraid and feels overwhelmed at times. When you're young, these feelings can be even stronger. Many of the young women who shared their experiences described feeling stupid and ashamed. *You are a good person.* This isn't a time to feel bad about yourself. You can't go back. You can't change what has happened. Wishing you had done something differently is wasted energy. You will need all your energy to make some important decisions. You have options to consider. You can embrace the decision-making process in a responsible way and choose what it is best for you, or you can decide not to, and accept whatever your parents or boyfriend encourage you to do. As Courtney advises, "making the best decision for yourself now is so important. It can be the foundation that will help you avoid, or maybe minimize, any feeling of self-doubt or regret later in life." The thought that you are responsible for making your decision is probably scary for you. You may be tempted to not make a decision. You can choose not to make a decision, but you must realize that choosing not to make a decision is a decision itself.

Deciding what you want to do about your pregnancy may be the biggest decision you've ever had to make. This is a big event in your life whether this is an unplanned or planned pregnancy. It may seem like you are faced with a monumental decision. This is normal. Many young women are overwhelmed at the thought of making this decision. You have options. You can continue your pregnancy and place your baby for adoption, or you can raise your baby. You can also choose to terminate your pregnancy. Many young women are aware that they have these options, yet they also know that no matter which option they choose, their life will be changed somehow. You may also be thinking this, and it is no doubt scary for you.

It may help you to know that you are not alone. Teenage pregnancy is not something new. Over the years, many young women have gotten pregnant when they didn't intend to, and have been faced with the same decision which you are about to make. Each year as many as one million teens become pregnant. The vast majority of these teens say they never intended to get pregnant. According to the Alan Guttmacher Institute, about half of all pregnant teens will choose to continue their pregnancies, slightly over one-third will choose to terminate their pregnancies, and the rest will end in miscarriage.* Only a few pregnant teens will choose to place their babies for adoption.

THINGS TO CONSIDER

- Before you go any further, take a deep breath and remember you are a special person. Your life is not over.
- Confirm your pregnancy. If you think you may be pregnant right now and you're not sure, don't waste any more time. Get a pregnancy test right away. If it's positive, see a health care provider. This does not lock you into continuing your pregnancy. You will need a physical

---

*A miscarriage occurs when, for some reason, the pregnancy does not develop normally and the mother's body expels the fetus before the baby is able to live outside the womb.

exam to determine how far along you are. This way you will know what your options are.

- Have confidence in yourself. Believe in yourself. You can make a good decision.
- Embrace the decision-making process. Learn as much as you can about all your options. This will help you make an informed decision and increase the likelihood that you will be content with whatever you decide to do.
- Reach out for help. Talk with your parent, guardian, and/or boyfriend. You may be afraid to tell your parents for any number of reasons. However, if you don't tell your parents, they may be very hurt and disappointed that you didn't share this with them, because chances are they will want to help you through your decision-making process. If you absolutely don't feel you can talk to your family, there are lots of other people who can help you. *Do not* make this decision alone. Here are just a few of the people you can talk to: school nurse, guidance counselor, favorite teacher, member of a religious group, youth group leader, family health care provider, mental health counselor, and/or counselor from a family planning clinic.
- Don't deny your pregnancy. You can't count on a miscarriage while you're making your decision. Also, there isn't anything you can do to end your pregnancy yourself. Anything your girlfriends might have told you about special drinks, bumpy roads, or anything else will not work. *You will only injure yourself.*

Your Options

Pregnancy is a major event in any woman's life, but especially in a young woman's life because so many areas of her life aren't settled yet. When most teens become pregnant they are still in school and financially dependent on a parent or guardian. Many teens are developing interests, and deciding what they want out of life. Making a decision about a pregnancy is a major event, especially at this stage in your life. Each option has its advantages and disadvantages. Each option brings with it a personal benefit or gain for you, as well as a personal loss. *No matter which option you choose, you can't escape a loss.* You will feel some pain from your loss and it will be necessary for you to grieve. Deciding when and whether to have a baby is a very personal decision. Only you know which option is best for you. The benefits and losses for each option will have a different meaning for each young woman. Carefully reviewing all your options will help you make the best possible decision for yourself.

LEGAL RIGHTS

Each option you have is a legal option. Legally you can choose to continue your pregnancy and raise your child, or you can place your child for adoption. Legally you can also choose to terminate your pregnancy. Many young women aren't aware of their legal rights. They don't realize they can get a pregnancy test, seek pregnancy counseling, have an abortion, or get prenatal care without informing their parents. This is a sensitive issue for some young women. They need to know their confidentiality will be maintained before they will seek care.

If you are a minor (under age eighteen) and living with your parents, your parents are responsible for you. As part of their responsibility, your parents' consent is required in most cases whenever you receive medical care and treatment. Parental consent laws vary in each state. In some states your health care provider may be required to inform one or both of your parents, and in other states one or both parents' consent is needed before medical care can be provided to you. However, there are times when your parents' notification or consent is not required.

Laws relating to health care for minors vary from state to state. Almost every state allows a minor to consent to the diagnosis and treatment of a sexually transmitted disease, as well as purchase nonprescription contraceptives, such as condoms. Most states also allow minors to consent to pregnancy-related care, which includes family planning and contraceptive services, prenatal care, delivery, and care after delivery.

As a minor, you can also get family planning services in federally funded programs without your parents' notification or consent. However, these programs are mandated to encourage parental involvement. This means these providers will encourage you to notify your parents and they may offer to speak to your parents with you. They will not do this unless they have your permission first, though. This is a difficult issue for some teens to talk to their parents about, and some teens appreciate their health care provider's support.

You have the legal right to an abortion; however, most states have parental notification or consent laws. This means that depending on which state you live in and your age, one or both of your parents, or your legal guardian, may need to be notified and/or give their permission before you can have an abortion. If states have these laws, they must provide a "judicial bypass." This gives you the opportunity to appear before a judge and try to demonstrate that you are mature enough to make your own decision without your parents' notification or consent.

Do not delay getting a pregnancy test or health care because you are concerned about confidentiality. You can increase your chances of having a healthy outcome, whether you decide to continue or terminate your pregnancy, by getting an early pregnancy test and getting early prenatal care or an early abortion. If you have concerns about confidentiality, ask your health care provider what her policy on confidentiality is. She should explain her policy to you, as well as be able to explain your state's laws. If you still have concerns, you can consult Planned Parenthood. You may be able to get additional information from your local legal aid office or another legal advocacy group. You can find the numbers to these organizations by looking up "Legal Services" in the Yellow Pages of your telephone directory.

Even though these are legal options, there may be practical restrictions which may make it difficult for you. For instance, even though you have the legal option to continue your pregnancy and get prenatal care, there are practical issues at stake. You will need to pay for your health care, and you'll need a place to live. If you're going to live at home, you'll have to work this out with your parents.

This is an important event in your life. We strongly encourage you to share this with your parent or guardian. They can provide you much-needed emotional support, as well as help you through the decision-making process. If you do not feel you can speak to your family, we strongly encourage you to speak with another older, responsible adult.

PARENTING

About half of the young women who become pregnant each year choose to raise their baby. You can raise your baby on your own or with the help and support of your family, your boyfriend, and/or others. You and your boyfriend can also marry, but few teens today choose to do this. According to statistics, of the teens who do marry, more than half of their marriages end in divorce.

Raising a baby is an awesome responsibility, even for women who are older when they become mothers. The lack of life experience, education, and financial security among teenagers makes it even harder for them to raise their children. Each teen parent has a different experience. Some teens meet the responsibility and challenge of parenting with strength and determination. Other teens become frustrated and overwhelmed with parenting. Lots of teens wished they had postponed parenting. As Sharon said:

> I love my daughter, yet there are times when I wish I had waited to have my baby. There is so much responsibility. There are so many things I worry about. There's never enough time in the day for me to do everything I need to do. I rush all day long. It begins early in the morning when I race around to get us both ready for school, and it seems like it never ends, especially on the nights when she doesn't sleep well.

Another teen, Kathy, said: "My son is great. I enjoy being a mother. I'm a good mother. I didn't know there was so much you had to do. Sometimes I think I would have been better off if I had put off having kids for a while. I grew up too fast. There are days when I feel so old, and I'm still just a kid."

Having a baby will drastically change your life. You will experience losses in many areas of your life. Your relationships will change with your family, your boyfriend, and other friends. You may have difficulty completing your education and you will probably struggle financially to make ends meet. Teen parenting has been linked with poverty. Teen moms do eventually catch up, but it takes them a very long time, and they will only make one-half the family income of their peers who postponed childbearing until their mid-twenties or later.

ABORTION

About one-third of all teens who become pregnant each year choose to terminate their pregnancy. For most teens, abortion is a personal, complex decision. Many teens carefully balance their religious or moral beliefs with their other needs when making their decision. Some women choose abortion even though it conflicts with their religious beliefs because they feel it is the best option for themselves. Other women don't choose abortion, either because they waited too long and it was no longer a possibility, or they can't resolve their religious or moral beliefs. There is an emotional loss associated with abortion. For each woman the emotional loss is different. As Jessica said:

> I'm not happy with myself that I had an abortion. It's against my religious views. But at the time there was too much going against me in my life. I

felt I did the responsible thing. It would have been too emotionally traumatic for me at that time to bring a child into this world.

ADOPTION

Monica chose to place her baby for adoption because she felt she wasn't ready to be a parent at the time and because she was morally opposed to abortion. Monica says:

> Abortion was never an option for me. I don't believe in abortion, although I wouldn't discourage another woman from having one if that's what she thought was best for her. I worked through the pros and cons of parenting versus adoption. For two months I wrote down how I felt about each option. Even though in the back of my mind I knew adoption was right for me, going through the process was very helpful. It made it concrete in my mind. It became very clear to me that adoption was the best decision I could make for my baby and myself.

Adoption is an option for a young woman, such as Monica, who feels she's not ready emotionally or financially to raise a child, and who does not feel comfortable terminating her pregnancy. There are many individuals and couples today who want to fulfill their dream of being parents. Adoptive children are raised in loving families. Some young teens do not choose adoption because they are worried that the emotional loss they would experience would be too great. A young woman who chooses adoption does experience the loss of parenting her baby. However, for the young women who choose adoption, this loss is not as great to them as the loss they believe they would have experienced if they had chosen either parenting or abortion. They want what's best for their baby, and they are concerned that at that point in their life they cannot be a good parent. Both Monica and Carolyn, who share their experiences in chapter 9, felt adoption was their best option. They are happy with their decision and do not have regrets. As Carolyn said:

> I didn't want to have an abortion. . . . I could have raised my child with my parents' support. But that wasn't what I wanted to do. I felt it wasn't fair for my child to grow up without a father. I wanted my child to have a better life than what I was able to give. I knew it would be hard for me to get my education. I wasn't emotionally ready to be a parent. The more I thought about it, adoption made the most sense.

Then and Now

Teen sex and teen pregnancy are not new. However, sexual activity begins at an earlier age for more young teens today than it did years ago. According to the Alan Guttmacher Institute, about 50 percent of the young women, and 75 percent of the young men today have sex before age eighteen, compared to 35 percent of young women and 55 percent of young men in the early 1970s. Young men and women also marry three to four years later today than teens did decades ago. In the past young teens did get pregnant outside of marriage, but it was handled much differently.

In the 1950s through the early 1970s when a young woman became pregnant she either married the man or secret arrangements were made to place her baby for adoption. Abortion was not legal until 1973. If a young woman wanted an abortion, she had to have an illegal one. Illegal abortions were associated with serious health risks. Some women died from them, and some women suffered serious medical complications. Fewer single women at that time raised their children alone. Society expected a young woman to marry or place her baby for adoption. Single women who raised their children were viewed as being less stable and more emotionally needy than the young women who placed their babies for adoption. There was a stigma attached to single parenting. It was considered socially unacceptable to be a young, single mother. Public assistance did not exist then for women who needed financial support so that they could stay at home to raise their children. Mosella was a single teenager when she became pregnant in 1955. She shares her experience so you can understand what women experienced in previous years:

> I was single and a teenager in 1955 when I became pregnant. That was over forty years ago and times have certainly changed since then. Back then, sex was only for married couples. It was something that happened behind closed doors. No one talked about sexuality. That was taboo. There was no sex education. It was almost impossible to get birth control. Women did not have careers; they married and had babies.
>
> If you were single and got pregnant your options were limited and bleak. You were expected to marry the father of your baby. Some women placed their babies for adoption and other women had illegal abortions. It didn't matter which option you chose. They were equally traumatic. If you planned to marry the man or to place your baby for adoption, you had to involve your family. This meant acknowledging to your family that you had had premarital sex. You got caught doing something you weren't sup-

posed to do. You were ashamed and felt guilty to have to tell or burden your family. You risked rejection by them and by society.

I never meant to get pregnant. I got caught. I felt very sad and guilty about my pregnancy. I didn't have anyone to talk to. There was no one I could trust. I was brought up in a strict family. My dad died when I was young. My brothers were brought up to be the head of the household. I couldn't face telling my family, so I made my decision alone.

At the time I got pregnant, I was one of the few colored women* attending a prominent music conservatory. I had worked very hard to be accepted to that school. I was awarded a full scholarship to attend. . . . That was something I was extremely proud of. My family and friends were also proud of me, and they had high hopes for me. I felt I couldn't disappoint them. I couldn't marry the father of my baby, and I couldn't place my baby for adoption. They did not have the type of adoption arrangements back then that they do today. My other two choices were to raise my baby alone or to have an abortion. I couldn't see bringing a child into this world. There weren't any good jobs then. I didn't know how I could manage, how I could be a good parent under those circumstances. My child would have lived in poverty, and that was not an option for me. I was determined to have a better life. Sure, I was spoiled. I wanted a taste of life. I wanted to experience life. It was not my mission to be a wife and mother. I was a dreamer. I had been given a chance of a lifetime. To be a colored woman attending a music conservatory was a very big opportunity for me. I wanted to fulfill a life dream. I wanted a career in music.

I chose to have an abortion. At first I tried to miscarry. But then I realized I didn't want to sacrifice my health. So I went out of town and had an abortion. I was very fortunate, my physical health was not harmed in any way. But I hurt emotionally. I'm Catholic, and so I felt very guilty about what I had done. For years, it was very hard for me to deal with because of my religion and also because I did everything alone. I never told anyone, so I suffered in silence. Twenty years later I finally told my family.

Who's to know whether I did the right thing? Who's to say? I feel I did the best thing for myself, and that's what counts. No one can judge me. I have healed since then. My faith in myself and in God saved me. Along the way I found help. Friends mentored me, they took an interest in me, they helped me reach my potential. I shared my feelings with a therapist. That also helped a lot. I've traveled to many places. I've lived a very rich and rewarding life. I have my master's degree in education and I have a career in music. I've fulfilled my dreams.

---

*This wording has been used at Mosella's request to reflect the terminology common at the time these events took place.

My advice to other teens is to trust someone. It's a big decision to make. Don't go through the decision process alone, like I did. Get proper counseling. No matter what you choose to do, take good care of your health. Today you can walk into any clinic and get good health care and be treated with dignity and respect. That's an option young women didn't have when I was a teenager. Above all else, have faith in yourself and in God that you will make the right decision. Take a chance on life. Do what you really want to do.

Mosella gives wonderful advice. She knows from her own experience how a young woman feels when faced with an unintended pregnancy. We are lucky today that many of the circumstances which made Mosella's experience difficult have changed. It was not legally possible for a single person to use prescriptive contraceptives such as the pill until 1972. Women did not have access to a safe, legal abortion until 1973. That wasn't all that long ago. In addition, it hasn't been socially acceptable to be a single parent until recent years.

Women have reproductive freedom today which years ago they didn't have. This freedom provides more options for a young woman, but it also carries with it responsibility. A young woman must decide for herself how she wants to resolve her pregnancy. Having more options doesn't necessarily make a decision easier; it means there are more decisions to make. In previous years it was socially unacceptable for a young, single woman to raise her baby alone. Today societal views toward teen pregnancy and parenting have changed. Although not everyone shares the same views, teen pregnancy and parenting does not carry the same level of shame it once did. There are some who still see it as a strictly moral issue, that teens should never participate in premarital sex, and these people may judge you for the choices you make. There are others who view parenting as a strictly economical issue. They resent and even protest against their tax dollars being spent to support unwed teens and their children. There are still others who have liberal views. They support and advocate programs to ensure that pregnant teens and their babies are adequately cared for. There is societal agreement about one thing, however, and that is responsibility. No matter which option a teen chooses, whether it is parenting, abortion, or adoption, society expects that she will be responsible. If she chooses to be a parent, it is expected that she will find the resources to support herself and her baby, and that she will continue with her education.

It is also acceptable for a young woman to choose not to be a parent. She can terminate her pregnancy or place her baby for adoption so that she can delay parenting until she is older, has had more life experiences, and feels ready to be a mother. Delaying parenting has its advantages. It gives a young woman the freedom while she is still young to learn more about herself, and to pursue other life goals without the burden of a child. Whereas in previous years young women tended to marry and have their babies at an earlier age, more young women today are living their lives differently. More young women are postponing childbearing until their mid-twenties or later so that they can have the freedom to get more education, travel, or gather other life experiences.

In the 1985 novel *In Country,* by Bobbie Ann Mason, Sam, a young woman, comments about the plight of her pregnant teen friend and says, "It used to be that getting pregnant when you weren't married ruined your life because of the disgrace; now it just ruined your life and nobody cared enough for it to be a disgrace."[3] Sara, the young woman at the beginning of this chapter, echoes a similar thought when she first finds out that she's pregnant. "How could I have let this happen? . . . What am I supposed to do now? My life is ruined." These young women are not alone in the way they think. Unfortunately, too many young women think that their lives are ruined because they are pregnant, and they give up their hopes and dreams. They think they won't be able to accomplish what they want to do. Your life is not ruined, it is not over. Today there are counseling services in place that are nonjudgmental which will help you explore all your options and help you select the one that's right for you. If you choose to raise your child, there are supportive services in place which will help you stay in school and help you to improve your life and the life of your child. There is no reason to give up hope or your dreams, no matter which option you choose. Dianne Wilkerson, the first African-American female state senator in Massachusetts, shares her personal experience in chapter 4. She offers this advice to pregnant teens:

> Feel good about yourself, feel good about your life and your goals. Don't give up on yourself. Your life is not over because you are pregnant. . . . Ask for help if you need it. When people see that you want to achieve they will help you.

This book will not tell you what to do. This book will provide you with facts on your options. Some of these facts you may already know; some of the facts you may not want to hear. Getting as many facts as you can about your options will help you choose what's best for you. The case studies provided will not give you all your answers, but perhaps you may see some of yourself in them. Some of the stories may seem repetitive, but the purpose is for you to sort things out and arrive at your own conclusions. You are the only person who knows what's right for you. What works for you may not work for someone else. Only you can decide what you want to do.

Notes

1. Bobbie Ann Mason, *In Country* (New York: Harper & Row, 1985).
2. The Alan Guttmacher Institute, "Teenage Reproductive Health in the United States," *Facts in Brief* (pamphlet), August 31, 1994.
3. Mason, *In Country,* p. 103.

2

Just the Facts

I didn't think it could happen to me . . .

"I thought it was one of my safe days, so I took the chance."

Dominique

"I trusted him, he told me it would be okay, he would withdraw in time."

Tara

"We had sex standing up; my girlfriends told me you couldn't get pregnant that way."

Margarita

"I thought I was too young. It was my first time. I'm only eleven years old."

Vivey

"I douched after we had sex. I thought that would wash away the sperm."

Lakeisha

A pregnancy begins when a man's sperm and a woman's egg join. The moment a sperm and egg unite a new life begins. This usually happens during sexual intercourse when a man ejaculates (releases) his sperm deep inside a woman's vagina, but a woman can also get pregnant even if she did not have sexual intercourse. If a man ejaculates near a woman's vagina, sperm can get into her vagina and travel up into the fallopian tube, where conception can occur. Most pregnancies, however, happen as a result of sexual intercourse. If you're going to have sex, it's best to always be careful and use contraception (a birth control method) correctly to avoid a pregnancy.

Some young women are tempted like Dominique was to try to prevent a pregnancy by avoiding sexual intercourse on days when they think they are fertile. This method of birth control is also known as natural family planning or the rhythm method. It's based on knowing a woman's reproductive cycle. Once a month a woman releases an egg, usually about two weeks before her next period is due. This is the time when a woman is most fertile. If sexual intercourse is avoided at this time a pregnancy generally will not happen. This method is not as easy as it seems. Young women typically have irregular periods, so there's no way of knowing for sure when the egg is released. Also, when an egg is released can be affected by emotions, stress, and nutrition. You are taking big chances if you rely on having sex only on your "safe days" to prevent a pregnancy. (Since the time of ovulation can be so unpredictable, even having intercourse around the time of your period can be risky.)

As Tara found out, the withdrawal method, when a man withdraws (pulls out) his penis from a woman's vagina before he ejaculates, is also risky and may not prevent a pregnancy. This method requires a great deal of self-control on the man's part. He must withdraw his penis before he ejaculates, or sperm can be left in a woman's vagina and she can become pregnant. However, sperm can be left in a woman's vagina even before a man withdraws his penis. This method is not reliable, and if a man is concentrating on when he ejaculates he probably is not enjoying sex as much. More important, having unprotected sexual intercourse is never a good idea. It puts both a man and a woman at risk for contracting a sexually transmitted disease (STD), as well as conceiving an unwanted pregnancy.

Margarita found out that standing up during sexual intercourse does not prevent a pregnancy. When sperm are deposited in the vagina they travel up, searching for a woman's egg. Sperm will always travel up, no matter which position you choose to have sex. Standing up or any other position during sexual intercourse will not prevent a pregnancy.

Young women, regardless of their age, can get pregnant before their first menstrual period. Vivey found this out. This is because a young woman begins ovulating before she has her period. Being young will not prevent you from becoming pregnant. Your body is already releasing eggs, and that's half of what it takes to become pregnant.

Some young women, like Lakeisha, believe they can prevent a pregnancy by douching after sexual intercourse. Douching, washing, or urinating after you have sex will not prevent a pregnancy. Douches or water cannot kill sperm. In fact, douching can even push the sperm up *toward* the uterus. Once a man ejaculates, his sperm reach the fallopian tube fairly quickly. This is why a contraceptive barrier such as a condom, for example, has to be in place before sexual intercourse begins in order for it to prevent a pregnancy.

Like these young women, a lot of teens have misconceptions about how to prevent a pregnancy. Many teens don't have a good understanding of the male and female reproductive systems. Misinformation can cause a lot of anxiety and fear. Most important, you can become pregnant when you do not want to.

In order to prevent a pregnancy, birth control needs to be used *each and every time* you have sexual intercourse or engage in very close sexual activity with a man. Birth control methods are designed to prevent a pregnancy. There are many different types of birth control. Some are more effective than others. Your health care provider can explain all of your options and help you select the method which is best for you. Usually you do not need your parents' permission to get birth control, although it's a good idea to discuss this with one of your parents or a responsible adult *before* becoming sexually involved with someone.

If you're thinking about taking your chances and not using birth control, here are some startling statistics which may change your mind:

- If you do not use birth control the first time you have sexual intercourse you are four times more likely to become pregnant than someone who uses birth control.
- One-half of all teen pregnancies happen within six months of the first sexual experience (losing your virginity).
- One-third of teen mothers have a second pregnancy within two years of their first baby.
- Each year three million teenagers will get an STD. Some STDs, like gonorrhea and chlamydia, can be cured, but if left untreated, they can lead to serious consequences, such as pelvic inflammatory disease (PID) and infertility. Others, like herpes or AIDS, have no cure, and you must live with them the rest of your life. Remember that if syphilis is left untreated, it can affect your brain and other organs and currently there is no cure for AIDS, which means you will die from it. STDs can be passed on to your baby during pregnancy and childbirth and can cause serious harm to your baby.

Reproductive Organs

FEMALE REPRODUCTIVE ORGANS

Your ability to reproduce or give birth to a baby occurs in cycles throughout your reproductive years. Each month changes occur within your body to prepare you for pregnancy. This is what's known as your menstrual cycle. As you grow up and mature you begin to ovulate, or release eggs. Once this happens you are able to conceive and give birth. A woman's reproductive ability begins around the time of her first menstrual cycle and generally ends when she no longer menstruates. A young woman first menstruates as early as age nine, or as late as age sixteen. Women stop menstruating at the time of menopause, which usually occurs when a woman is around fifty years old.

A woman's reproductive organs include her vagina, uterus (womb), two fallopian tubes ("egg ducts"), and two ovaries. The *vagina* is the tubular passageway connected to the uterus. During sexual intercourse, sperm enter the vagina and travel through the *cervix,* which is a very small opening at the neck of the uterus, into the uterus, and then into one of the fallopian tubes. You can see your vagina and feel your cervix, but the other female reproductive organs are not visible.

The *uterus* or womb is a muscular, pear-shaped organ in which a baby grows during pregnancy. Normally it is about the size of a fist. The uterus is located in your mid-pelvic area, behind your bladder and near your backbone. The inside walls of the uterus touch each other. During pregnancy the uterus expands and gets larger to make room for the growing fetus. At the base of the uterus is the cervix, the very small opening to the vagina. The cervix produces mucus which controls the flow of sperm into the uterus.

The *fallopian tubes* are connected on each side of the uppermost part of the uterus. The fallopian tubes are each about six inches long. They begin at the uterus and end near the ovary. The fallopian tubes are lined with cilia, which are tiny hair-like structures that move the egg to the uterus and the sperm from the uterus to the ovary.

The *ovaries* are small, almond shaped glands. Each woman has two ovaries. The ovaries have two very important functions: they produce the eggs and two female hormones important to reproduction. Each ovary lies just beneath the fallopian tube, about four or five inches below your waist. The ovaries are not attached to the fallopian tubes, but are kept in place by special tissue and body fat.

Fig 2.1: The Female Reproductive Organs

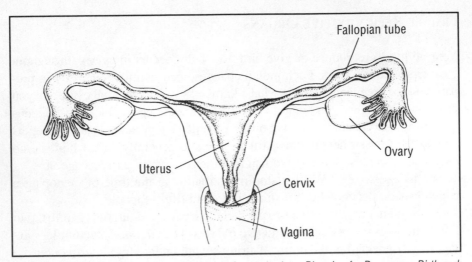

Source: American College of Obstetricians and Gynecologists, *Planning for Pregnancy, Birth and Beyond,* 2d ed. Washington, D.C.: ACOG, © 1995.

Figure 2.1 is a diagram of the female reproductive system. It shows where the organs are located in relation to each other.

MALE REPRODUCTIVE ORGANS

A man's reproductive ability is not limited like a woman's. Any time he produces sperm, if that sperm comes in contact with an egg, he is capable of fertilizing the egg, or in other words, getting a woman pregnant. Baby boys are born with many immature sperm cells. It is not until a young man reaches sexual maturity, which usually happens between the ages of thirteen and fifteen, that his sperm is capable of fertilizing an egg. While a woman's reproductive capability ends around the age of fifty, a man is capable of becoming a father well into his eighties.

A man's reproductive organs include his penis, testicles, and the ducts (tubes) which store and transport sperm. The penis and testicles are visible, while the sperm ducts are inside the body. The *testicles* hang below the penis. They are two reproductive glands which are located in a protective pouch called the *scrotum*. The sperm cells are produced in the man's testicles. When a man becomes sexually aroused sperm travel up the *sperm*

Fig 2.2: The Male Reproductive Organs

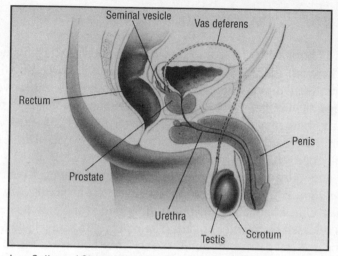

Source: American College of Obstetricians and Gynecologists, *Planning for Pregnancy, Birth and Beyond,* 2d ed. Washington, D.C.: ACOG, © 1995.

ducts, also called the *vas deferens,* over the bladder and through the prostate gland, where they mix with seminal fluid and then travel through the urethra, a tube which also carries urine away from the bladder and out of the body. (Both men and women have a urethra.) When a man has an orgasm he ejaculates the seminal fluid out of his *penis.* The amount of semen ejaculated equals about one-half to one teaspoon, but consists of about 500 million sperm. That's a lot of sperm at one time, which increases the risk of pregnancy that much more. This is nature's way of ensuring conception and thus the survival of the species. Roughly half of a man's sperm has defects which prevent them from fertilizing an egg. About 200 sperm actually reach the egg, but only one of them fertilizes the egg. Each sperm contains its own unique set of genetic material. This genetic material is how characteristics are passed from generation to generation. Each sperm is capable of creating an entirely different life with its own set of unique characteristics.

Figure 2.2 is a diagram of the male reproductive organs.

How Pregnancy Happens

REPRODUCTIVE CYCLE: OVULATION/MENSTRUATION

A woman is born with about five million egg cells already formed in the ovaries. These are all the egg cells that she will ever have. During the course of her reproductive years about 400 of these egg cells will develop into mature eggs. Nature has given a woman more than enough eggs necessary to conceive children; most egg cells are never used. Each egg cell is different from all the others. A baby born from one egg cell will be different from a baby born from any other egg cell.

Once a month an egg cell ripens and is released from the ovary. This is called *ovulation*. Normally ovulation alternates each month between your two ovaries. One month an egg is released by one ovary, and the next month the egg is released by the other ovary. The ripened egg travels down the fallopian tube and stays there for about twenty-four hours waiting to be fertilized by a man's sperm. Once the egg is released by the ovary the lining of the woman's uterus, the uterine lining, begins to build up so that it is prepared to receive the fertilized egg. If the egg is not fertilized by the man's sperm, then the egg disintegrates and is eliminated through the vagina. A woman is not even aware that this has happened. When a pregnancy does not take place, the lining of the uterus is no longer needed. It is shed or discarded during menstruation or what women refer to as their period.

Every month an egg is released by one of the ovaries, and every month the uterine lining is rebuilt to prepare for a possible pregnancy. The egg is usually released about two weeks before the next menstrual period. However, it's very difficult to know exactly when a young woman ovulates. If a pregnancy does not occur, the woman menstruates. Menstruation is the final phase of the hormonal changes known as the menstrual cycle which take place in a woman's body on a monthly basis. The cycle repeats over and over again from the time when a young woman first menstruates until later in her adult life when she reaches menopause and stops menstruating. In all, this will occur some four hundred times during a woman's reproductive years.

The average length of a menstrual cycle is twenty-eight days, but it can be as short as twenty days or as long as thirty-six days. Because the uterine lining is not discarded if pregnancy occurs, when a woman is pregnant she stops menstruating completely for nine months. A woman's menstrual cycle can stop for a short time or be late even when she's not pregnant. This can happen during stressful times, such as when there's a death in the family, if there's sickness in your family, if your family is planning on moving away, if you're worried about your school work, or if you're fighting with your best friend. Something minor like looking forward to a concert or a special outing can delay a menstrual cycle. Sometimes just worrying about whether or not you are pregnant can delay your menstrual cycle.

FERTILIZATION/CONCEPTION

As the egg travels down the fallopian tube it comes to a rest in the outer third portion of the tube. If the egg is met with sperm within twenty-four hours of ovulation a pregnancy can happen. Fertilization (or conception) occurs when the sperm and egg unite. The moment this happens a new life begins to form.

Sperm is deposited into the vagina by a man's penis during sexual intercourse. If the sperm is not blocked by a contraceptive (birth control method), the five hundred million sperm will make their way from the vagina through the cervical opening and through the woman's uterus and into her fallopian tube. Some of the sperm make their way very quickly and arrive at the fallopian tube within half an hour of sexual intercourse. Other sperm move very slowly and take several days to get to the fallopian tube. Sperm can survive for several days, which means that sperm may already be in the fallopian tube when the egg arrives. So even though an egg can only survive for twenty-four hours, a woman can still become pregnant if she has had sexual intercourse without using birth control within four or five days before ovulation. However, a woman is much more likely to become pregnant if she has sexual intercourse at the same time as she ovulates.

THE PROGRAMMING OF A NEW LIFE

After the egg has been fertilized by a sperm, the outer cell wall changes so that no other sperm can enter it. If another sperm entered the already fertilized egg, the development of the fertilized egg would stop. The pregnancy would not be able to continue. Thus, nature has a way of protecting itself by blocking out additional sperm.

The fertilized egg cell, which is also referred to as the zygote, has all the genetic material it needs. It has forty-six chromosomes, twenty-three from the egg, and twenty-three from the sperm. These chromosomes make sure that the baby will be unique, that it will be like no other human being alive.

When the egg and sperm fuse, the genetic blueprint for the developing baby has been programmed for life. The developing baby is either a boy or girl, will be short or tall, have brown or blond hair, curly or straight hair, and so on. This is because the chromosomes are made up of genes which contain all the hereditary characteristics which parents can pass on to their children. Each gene has a specialized code which tells the embryo, the developing baby, how to mature. For example, there is a code for hair color, eye color, height, sex, etc. Each parent contributes equally to this blueprint, but it is the sperm which determines whether the fertilized egg will become a boy or girl.

Although genes play an important role in determining your baby's health, how you care for yourself and your baby during pregnancy and after birth is equally important. Getting your baby off to a good start begins before he is born.

IMPLANTATION

Within twenty-four hours of conception the fertilized egg (zygote) begins to divide. The fertilized egg first divides into two cells, then four cells, then eight cells, then sixteen cells, and on and on. The fertilized egg stays in the fallopian tube for about three days after fertilization where it continues to divide and grow.

After that time the fertilized egg begins to make its way to the uterus. The fertilized egg, which is known as the blastocyst, must attach itself to the uterine lining if development of the pregnancy is to continue. The uterine lining is already prepared to receive the fertilized egg. However, the blastocyst is very selective. It takes several days to choose a site for implantation, although most blastocysts implant on the upper portion of the uterus. The blastocyst usually implants itself on the eighth day following fertilization. By this time the blastocyst consists of approximately two hundred cells. By the twelfth day after fertilization the blastocyst is securely attached to your uterine lining. By now the blastocyst consists of a couple thousand cells. The blastocyst remains implanted and continues to develop over the next nine months, first developing into an embryo, and then at eight weeks into the fetus.

Your Pregnancy

Your baby's life began when two separate cells joined together: one egg cell from you joined with one sperm cell from your baby's father. This fertilized

Fig 2.3: Ovulation

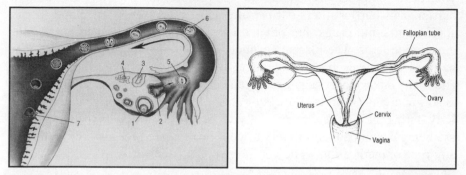

The egg matures in the follicle (1) and is released at ovulation (2). The follicle develops into the corpus luteum (3), which shrinks and disappears if pregnancy does not occur (4). If the egg (5) is fertilized by the sperm in the fallopian tube (6), it moves through the tube to the lining of the uterus (7), where it becomes implanted and grows.

Source: American College of Obstetricians and Gynecologists, *Planning for Pregnancy, Birth and Beyond,* 2d ed. Washington, D.C.: ACOG, © 1995.

egg cell is called the *zygote* and is the beginning of life. This cell will grow and develop inside your uterus over the course of nine months.

A normal pregnancy lasts about nine months. Your pregnancy began on the date of conception or fertilization (when the sperm and egg joined), and will continue until your baby is delivered. A pregnancy lasts about forty weeks from your last menstrual period and is divided into three time periods. Each time period is called a *trimester.* There are three trimesters in a pregnancy; each lasts about three months or twelve weeks.

During pregnancy your baby will grow inside your uterus, which will expand and make room for your developing baby. The inner wall of your uterus will thicken and the blood vessels will become bigger so that they can nourish your baby.

Your baby lives and grows inside the *amniotic sac* (also known as the bag of waters) and receives its nourishment from the *placenta.* The placenta starts to form the moment the fertilized egg attaches to your uterine wall. The baby is attached to the placenta by its umbilical cord. The placenta stays in place your entire pregnancy. It provides the lifeline by which oxygen and all the nutrients your fetus needs to grow and survive are passed from you to your fetus.

The placenta has many functions. In order for the embryo to continue to develop it needs nourishment, which the placenta brings from your blood to your developing baby. The placenta also protects the embryo by creating a barrier. This barrier filters out harmful substances from your blood. It can screen out some drugs, but other drugs pass through and can harm your developing fetus. The placenta cannot filter out alcohol, nicotine and other harmful substances in tobacco, illegal drugs such as cocaine and marijuana, and many other legal drugs which you can get at a drugstore. This is why it is so important not to take drugs or alcohol when you're pregnant, particularly during the first few months of your pregnancy when the baby's organs are being developed, and to talk to your health care provider before taking any type of medication while you're pregnant.

FIRST TRIMESTER

FETAL DEVELOPMENT

The first trimester is considered the first three months of pregnancy. Your developing baby is called an *embryo* for the first eight weeks; after that time until it is born it is called a *fetus*. In the first twelve weeks your fetus grows from just one fertilized cell to thousands of cells measuring three inches long and weighing about an ounce. This is an important time in your baby's development, as all the major organs are being formed. Your growing baby is particularly vulnerable during this time. Your fetus can be harmed by certain illnesses you may get and by drugs, including nicotine or alcohol that you use. As soon as you suspect that you might be pregnant you should stop drinking alcohol and using any drugs. You should contact your health care provider before you take any medications.

The baby's heart, lungs, brain, and other organ systems begin to develop during the first three months of your pregnancy. Your baby's heart will start to beat by the twenty-fifth day of your pregnancy, but may not be heard before the fourteenth week of your pregnancy. By the end of the first trimester your baby will be a fetus that is completely formed.

Figure 2.4 shows what your baby looks like at various stages throughout your pregnancy.

YOUR DEVELOPMENT

Some women know they are pregnant within one to two weeks after conception. A missed menstrual period may be the first sign that you are preg-

Fig 2.4: The Growth and Development of the Fetus

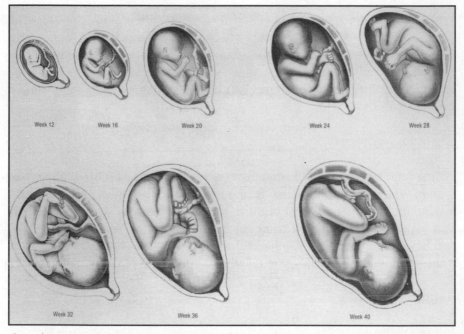

Source: American College of Obstetricians and Gynecologists, *Planning for Pregnancy, Birth and Beyond,* 2d ed. Washington, D.C.: ACOG, © 1995.

nant. You may also experience other signs of pregnancy: nausea, with or without vomiting; swollen, tender breasts; urinating more frequently; and feeling more tired than usual. You may be surprised to find out you're pregnant, and may experience some anxiety about this. You will probably not gain much weight during this trimester.

SECOND TRIMESTER

FETAL DEVELOPMENT

The middle three months mark the second trimester of your pregnancy. The fetus grows rapidly during this time. The fetus increases its activity all during this trimester, and exercises by kicking, stretching, and doing somersaults.

YOUR DEVELOPMENT

As the fetus grows you will become more aware of the new life within your womb. You can feel the first fetal movement, known as "quickening," around the fifth month. Most of the unpleasant pregnancy symptoms which you experienced in the first trimester have gone away. You will feel good, and have more energy. If you haven't made a decision about what you plan to do about your pregnancy you may be feeling more anxious and stressed.

THIRD TRIMESTER

FETAL DEVELOPMENT

The last three months are considered the third (and final) trimester of pregnancy. This time period is one of tremendous growth. The fetus gains most of its weight now, particularly during the ninth month. At the beginning of the third trimester, the fetus weighs about one and a half pounds and is almost twelve inches long. By the end of this trimester the fetus weighs between six and a half to seven and a half pounds and is about nineteen inches long. Some very important events occur throughout this entire trimester which are important for your baby's health and survival. Babies born after thirty-seven weeks are considered full term and ready to safely live outside the mother's uterus. After the thirty-seventh week of pregnancy, the lungs are mature and able to work outside of the mother's uterus. The brain continues to develop all during this trimester and after birth. The fetus also receives antibodies (proteins) from you which help it fight off infection for several months after birth.

YOUR DEVELOPMENT

Your baby gains most of its weight now, and you will also gain weight. You will look pregnant. People may comment about your pregnancy, and ask you questions like "When will your baby be born?" Because you get bigger as your fetus grows, you may find it difficult to move around. Your posture will change as your fetus grows and you may have backaches, and you will tire easily. The growing fetus puts extra pressure on your bladder, so you will have to urinate more frequently. Your hands and feet may swell, and you might have leg cramps, especially at night. You may also experience mood swings, from being excited about seeing your baby soon to being grumpy because of the common aches and pains you experience at this stage in your pregnancy.

SIGNS OF PREGNANCY

The first sign that a woman is pregnant is usually a missed menstrual period. This happens because very early on the placenta notifies the ovaries that the woman is pregnant. The ovaries stop releasing an egg every month, and the woman no longer menstruates. The placenta also begins to produce two hormones: progesterone and human chorionic gonadotropin (HCG). A pregnancy test looks for HCG levels to determine if a woman is pregnant.* It is the rapid rise in these two hormonal levels which cause the unpleasant side effects you may experience during their first trimester. These hormonal levels decrease at the beginning of the second trimester which is why many of these symptoms go away as the pregnancy progresses.

Some women may experience some pregnancy symptoms before they miss a period. These early pregnancy symptoms include swollen, tender breasts, nausea with or without vomiting (also known as "morning sickness" because it typically happens early in the day, but it can also happen any time during the day, and can be triggered by certain odors), urinating more frequently, tiring easily, and having difficulty concentrating.

Many pregnant women experience these symptoms during the first

---

*Pregnancy tests will be discussed in more detail later in this chapter.

trimester of their pregnancies. Some pregnant women experience all of these symptoms, and some experience only some of these symptoms. For instance, about half of all pregnant women experience nausea and vomiting, the other half do not. It's best to have a pregnancy test immediately if you have had sexual intercourse without adequate birth control and you are experiencing any of these symptoms, because you may be pregnant. *You may not experience all of these symptoms when you are pregnant.*

COMMON SIGNS OF PREGNANCY

- One or more missed menstrual periods
- Nausea/vomiting ("morning sickness")
- Swollen, tender breasts
- Urinating frequently; and
- Feeling more tired than usual

PREGNANCY TESTS

Pregnancy tests look for the placental hormone HCG in a woman's blood or urine. A positive pregnancy test almost always means that you are pregnant. However, if your pregnancy test is negative, that does not necessarily mean that you are not pregnant. Sometimes you can get a false negative test, which means the test result is negative even though you are pregnant. A false negative test can happen for any number of reasons including that the test was done too soon; the urine sample you used was not the first sample in the morning or it was contaminated; or you may have an abnormal pregnancy, such as an ectopic or tubal pregnancy or one you are about to miscarry.

WHERE TO GET A PREGNANCY TEST

You can have a blood or urine test done at a family planning clinic (for example, Planned Parenthood), at an adolescent clinic at your local hospital, or by a health care provider (doctor, midwife, nurse practitioner, physician's assistant). You may opt to test your own urine using a home pregnancy kit which you can purchase from a drugstore.

Lab Tests. A standard urine laboratory test done at a clinic or by your health care provider will usually be able to detect if you are pregnant around the time of your missed period. Getting a lab pregnancy test has its advantages. You may find out sooner if you're pregnant than you would if you tested your urine at home. Finding out that you're pregnant at an early stage in your pregnancy is very important. If you know you are pregnant you can begin making decisions about your pregnancy, giving you more options. If you go to your health care provider or family planning clinic you will get your results back from someone who can counsel you on all your available options.

Home Pregnancy Test. A home pregnancy test offers the advantage of being convenient, however, it is not as accurate as a lab test. This means it may not determine if you are pregnant until a week or so after you have missed your menstrual period. If you do use a home pregnancy test it is important to follow the directions very carefully. One disadvantage of a home pregnancy test is that you will be alone when you get the results, and this could be scary for you. If the test is positive you need to have a physical exam with a clinician as soon as possible. This will determine how far along you are in your pregnancy and what your due date will be. If the test is negative, you may still be pregnant. Remember, a false negative test can happen even if you are pregnant. If the test is negative and you are experiencing pregnancy symptoms you should have a repeat pregnancy test done by a clinic or clinician as soon as possible. *Do not wait hoping you will get your period. You may need medical attention.*

DELIVERY DATE

To determine your estimated due date the following formula is used: starting on the *first* day of your *last* menstrual period, add seven days and count back three months. For example:

First day of last menstrual period (LMP)	April 15
Add seven days	+ 7 days
	April 22
Subtract three months	– 3 months
Estimated delivery date (Due Date)	January 22

This method gives you and your health care provider a rough idea of the date your baby will be born. This method is not entirely accurate. It is more likely to be accurate if your menstrual cycles are regular and last twenty-eight days. Many young women have irregular menstrual cycles, and are unsure of the exact date of their last menstrual period.

In order to more accurately predict your delivery date, your health care provider will do a pregnancy test and an internal pelvic exam. An internal pelvic exam is done to confirm pregnancy and measure the size of your uterus. At each stage in your pregnancy, your uterus will be a different size. If done in the first trimester of pregnancy, an internal pelvic exam and the estimated delivery date will give you and your health care provider the most likely date your baby will be born.

Your due date is an important piece of information to know. It lets you know how far along you are in your pregnancy so that you can begin to make important decisions about what you want to do. Should you continue with your pregnancy, your health care provider will use your due date to monitor your baby's growth. This way you will know if your baby is growing normally. Your health care provider will also be able to screen or look for medical complications and be better able to take care of you and your baby.

Medical Problems during Pregnancy

Most women do not experience serious medical problems during their pregnancies. Women who are in good health before they get pregnant, who take good care of themselves while they are pregnant, and who get adequate prenatal care do not experience medical problems as often during their pregnancies as women who do not do these things. Women who are very young and who are older tend to experience more medical problems during their pregnancies. Researchers who have been studying the effects of age on pregnancy have found that it's not young age which puts teens at risk. Instead it's other factors, such as not getting adequate health care during pregnancy, poor nutrition, smoking cigarettes, drinking alcohol, using illegal drugs, or taking medications that may be harmful which put teens at risk for developing serious complications during their pregnancy. By taking good care of yourself during your pregnancy, getting regular health care, and maintaining a healthy lifestyle you can reduce the chance of medical complications during pregnancy and increase your chances of delivering a healthy baby.

COMMON MEDICAL COMPLICATIONS
AMONG PREGNANT TEENAGERS

- Anemia
- Pregnancy Induced Hypertension
- Preterm Labor

According to the American College of Obstetricians and Gynecologists (ACOG) these complications, each of which will be explained in detail, are even more common for pregnant teens who are less than fifteen years of age.

EARLY PREGNANCY

All pregnant women are at risk of developing complications early in their pregnancy. During the first months of pregnancy you can have an ectopic (tubal) pregnancy or a miscarriage. These are serious conditions which require immediate medical attention. This is one of the reasons why it is so important for you to get early and regular prenatal care when you think you are pregnant.

ECTOPIC PREGNANCY

In a normal pregnancy, a fertilized egg travels down the fallopian tube and implants itself in the uterine wall. In some pregnancies, as the fertilized egg travels down the fallopian tube on its way to the uterus something goes wrong. Sometimes the fertilized egg remains in the fallopian tube. If the fertilized egg attaches itself to the wall of the fallopian tube, an ectopic (tubal) pregnancy can result. At first you may feel early signs of pregnancy, such as a missed menstrual period, nausea and vomiting, or breast tenderness. As the growing embryo runs out of room, the tube may rupture (burst open). If this happens you will experience sharp, intense lower abdominal pain which is usually one-sided. You may also have irregular vaginal bleeding. *This is a medical emergency and requires immediate medical attention.* Not obtaining medical attention at this time could put your life in danger. The number of ectopic pregnancies has been increasing in recent years. Tubal damage caused by a sexually transmitted disease which is not adequately treated puts you at an increased risk for an ectopic pregnancy. Tubal damage affects your future fertility, which can make it that much more difficult for you to become pregnant.

WARNING SIGNS

- Sudden, sharp lower abdominal pain, usually on one side
- Irregular vaginal bleeding with abdominal pain when your period is late or has been abnormally light
- Episodes of feeling faint or dizzy[1]

A woman experiencing these symptoms should seek immediate medical attention.

MISCARRIAGES

At least 15 percent of all pregnancies miscarry in the first trimester. A miscarriage usually happens because there is something wrong with the developing pregnancy. When you miscarry you lose your baby. Usually there is nothing you could have done to prevent the miscarriage.

Heavy vaginal bleeding along with abdominal cramps and a backache are the usual signs of a miscarriage. If vaginal bleeding continues it may be necessary for your doctor to do a surgical procedure called dilation and curettage (D&C). This will empty your uterus, stopping your bleeding and cramping. This procedure is not always needed, though.

WARNING SIGNS

- Heavy bleeding, possibly with clots of tissue, and cramping or a backache
- Abdominal pain and/or fever[2]

A woman experiencing these symptoms should seek immediate medical attention.

THROUGHOUT YOUR PREGNANCY

ANEMIA

Your body requires extra iron during pregnancy. The extra iron is needed for your developing baby. Many teens already suffer from anemia (also known as iron-poor blood) because of poor eating habits. Your health care provider may want you to take extra iron. Eating well-balanced meals which include foods rich or high in iron (such as liver, spinach, greens, and beans) will help increase your iron stores. If you become anemic you may feel tired during your pregnancy and you will not be in the best condition to enter labor. In addition, to be healthy and to grow properly your developing baby needs iron.

SEXUALLY TRANSMITTED DISEASES

Sexually transmitted diseases are infections which you get when you have unprotected sexual intercourse with an infected partner. Some STDs, like gonorrhea and chlamydia, can be treated and cured. Other STDs, such as AIDS and herpes, can't be cured; only the symptoms can be treated. This means you live with these infections for the rest of your life, and you can pass these infections to other sexual partners and to your baby during pregnancy and childbirth. It's very important to follow your health care provider's instructions for treatment of an STD during pregnancy. This may prevent you from passing the STD to your baby during childbirth. Table 2.1 lists various STDs and the effects they can have on you and your unborn baby.

Gonorrhea and chlamydia infections are the two most common STDs in adolescents. If you have a chlamydial infection during pregnancy which is not treated, your baby can be born too early. If this happens your baby is at an increased risk for serious medical problems such as lung, digestive, or neurological (brain) problems. Chlamydia can also cause pneumonia and eye infections in newborn babies. Gonorrhea can also cause serious eye infections in newborns and both it and chlamydia can be passed on to your baby during childbirth.

LATER PREGNANCY

PREGNANCY INDUCED HYPERTENSION

Pregnancy induced hypertension (PIH, also known as preeclampsia) is another medical complication of pregnancy which is common among pregnant adolescents. PIH is a condition which can begin around your fifth month of pregnancy. The condition may be mild or severe. The most common signs you may experience are high blood pressure and edema (swelling). Your health care provider will monitor your pregnancy very closely for signs of this illness, such as high blood pressure or protein in your urine. One of the dangers of this disease is that you may feel fine and actually be very sick. Regular prenatal care will make sure that this condition is picked up at an early stage, so that it can be monitored and treated. If PIH becomes severe and if it's not treated, it can be dangerous or life-threatening for you and your baby. If the condition becomes very severe, your baby may have to be delivered early.

Table 2.1: How Sexually Transmitted Diseases Can Affect You and Your Baby

Disease	Symptoms in Women	Effects on	
		Mother	Fetus/Baby
AIDS*	Appetite or weight loss, fatigue, swollen lymph nodes, night sweats, fever or chills, persistent diarrhea or cough; may have no symptoms	Immune system damage, leading to infections (such as pneumonia) or cancers; death	Immune system damage leading to death in 3 years in most infants
Chlamydia	Vaginal discharge, painful or frequent urination, pelvic pain; may be no symptoms	Pelvic inflammatory disease, ectopic pregnancy	Eye infection, pneumonia
Genital herpes	Flulike symptoms (fever, chills, muscle aches, etc.); small, painful, fluid-filled blisters on genitals or buttocks	Recurrent outbreaks	Severe skin infection, nervous system damage, blindness, mental retardation, death
Genital warts	Possible genital itching, irritation, or bleeding; warts may appear as small, cauliflower-shaped clusters	Warts grow in size and number; may have abnormal Pap test	Warts on the vocal cords in early adolescence
Gonorrhea	Vaginal discharge; minor genital irritation, pain and fever; most women have no symptoms	Pelvic inflammatory disease, arthritis	Eye infection if left untreated
Syphilis	A painless open sore called a chancre; later rash, sluggishness, or slight fever	Damage to heart, blood vessels, and nervous system; blindness, insanity, death	Miscarriage, stillbirth, syphilis in liveborn infant

*AIDS stands for acquired immunodeficiency syndrome.

Source: American College of Obstetricians and Gynecologists, *Planning for Pregnancy, Birth and Beyond,* 2d ed. Washington, D.C.: ACOG, © 1995.

PRETERM LABOR

Young teens are at risk of delivering their babies too early, and this risk is even greater for teens who are less than fifteen years old. Babies delivered prematurely (too early) have an increased risk of developing serious medical problems. This is because a baby born too early is not fully grown and is usually underweight (also referred to as a low-birthweight baby, this is a baby that weighs less than five and a half pounds). Full-term babies may also be born underweight if for some reason their growth was slowed while they were still in their mother's womb. Low-birthweight babies are more likely than normal birthweight babies to suffer medical problems and to die in their first few months of life. Because they are so small, many of these babies require special medical care and can be sick or hospitalized for many months. Getting early and regular prenatal care as well as maintaining a healthy lifestyle, such as eating nutritious meals, gaining an adequate amount of weight, reducing stress, and getting the right amount of rest and exercise increases your chances of delivering a healthy, full-term baby.

Emotional Responses Associated with Pregnancy

Pregnancy is a major event, a developmental milestone, in any woman's life. Every woman experiences highs, such as joy and excitement, and lows, such as stress and anxiety. Pregnancy not only confirms your biologic capability to bring a child into this world, it also challenges every aspect of your entire being. Pregnancy will challenge you physically, emotionally, and intellectually. Your adjustment to pregnancy, whether or not your pregnancy was planned, can be very challenging because being pregnant and having a baby at this point in your life forces you to assume adult roles and behaviors which you may not be ready for. You probably have not finished high school, and still depend on your parents or guardians to pay for housing, clothing, food, etc. This is a time in your life when your main focus is developing yourself, finding out what your interests are and developing friendships. Right now you are probably relying on your friends and family for emotional support. Usually at this time you are not responsible for anyone but yourself. Having a baby forces you to be responsible and make major decisions before you may want to.

Physically your body will undergo many changes as you gain the average twenty-five to thirty pounds in pregnancy. Each trimester your body will change and you will feel different physically. There are some important questions to ask yourself: "Do I want to subject myself right now to a pregnancy?" "Can I deal with the change in my physical appearance?" and "How will this pregnancy have an impact on my overall physical well-being?" This last question is especially important if you already have a medical condition such as diabetes. You need to talk this over with your health care provider to help you determine what, if any, the additional medical risks of your pregnancy are. In this way you can decide if you want to take these risks.

Emotionally you must prepare yourself for the realities of motherhood. Again, there are some tough questions to ask yourself: "Am I emotionally ready to be a mother?" "Is this the right time in my life?" and "Am I prepared for the changes which will occur in my lifestyle, and with the important relationships in my life, such as with my boyfriend, family, and friends?" Whether your pregnancy was planned or unplanned it is a major life event. You will experience a range of emotions which will change as your pregnancy progresses.

Intellectually you must determine what your new needs will be. You should spend some time learning about and planning for these needs. Ask yourself: "Can I afford to have a baby now?" "Do I have adequate health care insurance?" "Will I be able to support myself and my baby when I am no longer living with my parents?"

You will no doubt spend a lot of time making your decision about what to do about your pregnancy. You will probably ask yourself these questions and more. This is an important decision with a big impact on your life now and in the future. An important decision like this requires time and thoughtful analysis.

When you choose to be a mother or place your baby for adoption, you are choosing to bring a life into this world. With either of these two choices comes a lot of responsibility. You have a big job ahead of you. Your goal is to have a healthy baby and remain healthy yourself. During each trimester of pregnancy there is an important task which you need to accomplish to achieve your goal. Recognizing your emotions and managing them will help you with these tasks. Your emotional health is just as important as your physical health; in fact, your emotional well being can have a major impact on how you feel physically during your pregnancy, on how you cope, and ultimately on the health of your baby.

FIRST TRIMESTER

YOUR FEELINGS

Most young women respond to the news of their pregnancies with a mix of feelings. Some are happy and excited and even feel a sense of power at being able to create a new life, while others feel sadness and anxiety about what their life and their baby's life will be like. A lot of young women want families, but they feel their pregnancy happened at the wrong time. Many others describe emotions such as shock, anger, disappointment in themselves or their boyfriend, and fears of rejection by their boyfriend, parents, or friends. These feelings are all normal. A lot of women experience these feelings no matter what their age. They can cause a great deal of distress, especially because they come at a time when you are probably not feeling physically well, as you may be experiencing some of the common discomforts of early pregnancy. The way you respond to or cope with these feelings is what's important. If you are continuing your pregnancy it is essential to be aware of and deal with these feelings.

PREGNANCY TASK

It's essential for your health and your baby's health whether you parent or place your baby for adoption to get early and regular care throughout your pregnancy. This means you start prenatal care during the first trimester and see your clinician regularly throughout the pregnancy.

Positive Ways to Cope

- Begin prenatal care with a health care provider you trust. Bring someone supportive with you to your appointments, such as your boyfriend, parent, or friend. Involving someone who cares about you will help you stay focused and motivated to take very good care of yourself.
- Adopt a healthier lifestyle. *Do not smoke cigarettes, drink alcohol, or take drugs or medications unless directed by your health care provider.*
- Improve your diet. Feed your growing baby foods which will help him grow. Eat three well-balanced, nutritious meals a day from all five food groups: grain products, vegetables, fruits, milk and milk products, and meat or other foods high in protein. Drink plenty of fluids such as milk, water, and 100 percent fruit juice throughout the day. Cut back on snacks and fatty foods which have limited nutritional value.
- Enjoy regular exercise. Usually you can participate in moderate exercise. Speak to your health care provider about what is appropriate for you and your baby at this stage of your pregnancy.
- Know your options. If you honestly feel that you are not ready or prepared for pregnancy or parenthood right now, you do have options. You can safely have an abortion during the first trimester. You can also consider

placing your baby for adoption. Discuss your feelings about your options with someone you can trust, such as a parent, a guardian, an older friend who knows what you're going through, or a counselor.

- Be good to yourself. Now is not the time to be hard on yourself. You're not alone. Other teens have also become pregnant when they didn't intend to. Right now you need all your energy to focus on what is best for you and your baby. Stay in school. Continue other activities in your life which are important to you. Consider joining a teen parent group for peer support.

SECOND TRIMESTER

YOUR FEELINGS

Many young women are just now starting to get prenatal care. They didn't start prenatal care in the first trimester for lots of different reasons, usually because they hadn't acknowledged they were pregnant, or they didn't know where to get prenatal care, or were afraid to get prenatal care. The fetus moves for the first time usually during the fifth month. This fetal movement reinforces the reality of future parenthood. This may be exciting for you if you are happy about your pregnancy. It may be scary if you are concerned about becoming a mother or if you have decided to place your baby for adoption. The fetus is growing rapidly during the second trimester, and you are too. You can no longer hide your pregnancy. You will now need to wear maternity or baggier, looser-fitting clothes. Some young women like the changes in their bodies and feel attractive; others are bothered by the weight gain and feel very self-conscious.

PREGNANCY TASK

Understand that your fetus is a developing baby with its own needs, yet still dependent on you to nourish it. It's essential that you take very good care of your developing baby. You do this by taking very good care of yourself.

Positive Ways to Cope

- Continue getting prenatal care. Communicate any fears and/or concerns you may have with your health care provider. She can better help you if she knows what you're feeling. She can also help by referring you to community resources you may need.

- Continue healthy lifestyle changes. *Do not drink alcohol, smoke ciga-rettes, take drugs, or use medications unless directed by your health care provider.*
- Continue healthy eating habits. This is not the time to try to diet. Your health care provider can refer you to a nutritionist if you're concerned you may be gaining too much weight. A nutritionist can help you plan healthy, well-balanced meals, as well as let you know if your weight gain is too little or too much.
- Continue regular exercise. Some exercise is good for you now. It can help you feel better emotionally. It can also help relieve pregnancy discomforts such as backaches. Speak to your health care provider about what is appropriate for you and your baby at this stage of your pregnancy.
- If you feel uncomfortable at your school, consider switching to an alter-native high school for pregnant teens. Your guidance counselor can help you with this process.
- Be good to yourself. If you have decided to continue with your pregnancy whether you will parent or place your baby for adoption, you need to take very good care of yourself. Your baby's health depends on your health while you are pregnant. Talk about your feelings with someone you trust. Meet regularly with a teen support group. Discussing your feelings with other teens who are in the same situation will help. Continue with your education. Continue with the other activities in your life which are impor-tant to you.
- Explore all your options if you feel you may not be ready to be a parent. An abortion done now has more medical risks than if done in the first trimester. Talk to your health care provider. You may still be able to have an abortion. Your health care provider will let you know what the medical risks are, and where you can go. She can refer you to a social worker if you're having trouble finding the money to pay for an abortion. Consider adoption. You can do this by talking to an adoption agency, other teens who have placed their babies for adoption, or adoptive parents. Consid-ering adoption now does not mean you have to choose this option. It may help you to feel better about what you want to do. If you're having doubts about being a mother don't get wrapped up in preparing the nursery. This may only increase your anxiety, and lock you into being a mother before you've decided that's what you want to do. Explore all your options first. There is plenty of time in the third trimester to buy things for the baby.

THIRD TRIMESTER

As the final trimester progresses it's common to want the pregnancy to be over. The physical discomforts of the advancing pregnancy, such as backaches, leg cramps, urinating more frequently, feeling tired and achy may be taking an emotional toll on you. You may have fears and anxiety about labor and the birth of your baby. These are normal and may be increased because you might not have ever been in a hospital before and don't know what to expect. You may be afraid of childbirth. You may have heard horror stories about someone's long, painful labor. Many women dream about childbirth and their babies now. Nightmares are not unusual. Talk to a childbirth educator so that you will know what to expect. Concerns about being a good mother as well as unresolved problems with your own mother or your baby's father may arise. This is normal. As childbirth approaches, everyone's roles change. You may not feel you're getting the support you need from your boyfriend or your parents. Your boyfriend may be just as confused and scared about childbirth as you are. Your parents may be wondering how they will be able to find the time to help you as well as work and continue with their other obligations. If you've chosen to place your baby for adoption, you may be having some anxiety wondering what the hospital experience will be like.

PREGNANCY TASK

Giving birth is just around the corner. This is the time you often begin to identify yourself as a mother, and start feeling loving and nurturing toward your baby. It's also important to set realistic expectations for the demands of parenting.

Positive Ways to Cope

- Continue getting prenatal care. Follow the advice of your health care provider.
- Continue healthy lifestyle changes. Your baby's brain is growing now. You do not want to do anything which will harm his brain growth. *Do not drink alcohol, smoke cigarettes, take drugs, or use medications unless directed by your health care provider.*
- Continue regular exercise. The added weight you have gained may make

it harder, but it's not impossible to get some exercise. Light exercise will help with fatigue and backache. It's especially important to discuss with your health care provider what exercises or activities are safe to do now.

- Participate in childbirth classes. This will prepare you for labor and help you feel less frightened and more relaxed when labor begins.
- Continue to explore adoption if you feel you may not be emotionally ready to be a parent.
- If you're planning on placing your baby for adoption, talk about your feelings with someone you trust. Make a plan for labor and your hospital birth experience.
- Begin preparing for the baby. If you've decided to parent, now is the time to prepare the nursery. It's important to find day care. Your school may be able to help you find day care on site or in your community. Perhaps a neighbor or family relative may agree to babysit.
- Be good to yourself. With your advancing pregnancy you are probably experiencing intense emotions. Take good care of your physical and emotional health. Your baby's health depends on you. Continue with your education. If you can no longer go to school, your guidance counselor will help arrange for a home tutor.
- Talk your feelings over with someone you trust. Remember, these emotions are a normal part of pregnancy.

Notes

1. Robert A. Hatcher et al., *Contraceptive Technology*, 16th rev. ed. (New York: Irvington Publishers, Inc., 1994), p. 466.

2. Ibid.

3

Deciding What's Right for Me

In the middle of difficulty lies opportunity.

Albert Einstein

Sara was having difficulty concentrating in school. She wished she could hide until she figured out what she was going to do. At first she was successful at doing that. She stayed home sick for two days, faking the flu. But that morning her mother informed her she would have to go to school, or go to the doctor's office. She had no other choice. Going to the doctor with her mom was one of the last things she wanted to do. Sara found herself crying in the middle of class, and walking around the hallways in a daze. Her best friend, Jane, asked her if she was okay. Sara shrugged her shoulders, and told her she was still not feeling well. Sara knew she had a big decision to make. She knew she had to talk to someone soon. She just wasn't sure where to start.

The idea of being pregnant is initially terrifying to many young women. Feelings of guilt, shame, sadness, fear, and other emotions can be overwhelming. These emotions can be crippling at first, immobilizing a young woman in such a way that she doesn't know what to do. Suddenly a young woman finds herself faced with a major decision to make, and she's not sure which way to turn or who to trust.

When an unexpected event happens in our life we often react with shock and disbelief. There's a tendency to want to protect ourselves from what we fear could be further harm. Like Sara, you may want to cocoon yourself for a while, curl up into a ball and shelter yourself until the shock passes. Sometimes it can help, giving you a chance to regroup, so you have the energy you need to make your decision. Other times it doesn't help. Valuable time and energy are wasted worrying about something which you can't change. Sara stayed home at first, but it didn't help much. She spent the time worrying about what she was going to do. She had to go back to school. At school she felt distracted and had difficulty concentrating. The pressure to do something didn't go away. She knew she needed to do something. She wasn't sure what, and she struggled, not knowing where to begin.

An unintended pregnancy can be very scary at any age. Deciding when and whether to have a baby is a deeply personal and complex decision. This decision may seem enormous to you, and you may be frightened by the idea of making it. This may be the first big decision you've ever made. There's probably a lot going through your mind now. You may be wondering how your life will change. You may be unsure if you're ready to have a baby yet. You may also be worried that you won't have any control in making your decision. This is a very big decision to make, but *it's a decision that you are capable of making*. It's normal to feel vulnerable, to have some self-doubts. When we are faced with difficult situations like this, we're challenged. As we work through these challenges we learn more about ourselves, and we grow from them. *In the middle of difficulty lies opportunity*. This is an opportunity for you to learn more about yourself, to clarify your values, and to shape your life in the direction you want to go.

Each young woman's reaction to her pregnancy is different. The vast majority of teens say they didn't intend to get pregnant, so this is a scary time for them. There are, however, some young women who wanted to get pregnant and planned their pregnancies. These young women feel they're ready to be mothers at this time in their life. Here's what Barbara says:

> I was excited to find out that I was pregnant. I felt powerful. My boyfriend and I created a life. I'm holding this life inside me. My boyfriend and I planned it this way. We just graduated from high school. We're eighteen. We plan on marrying after the baby is born. Our life goal is to be together and have a family. We very much want our families' support. Even though we're certain about what we're doing, we're nervous about telling our families. We're not sure how they will react.

Whether your pregnancy is unintended or intended you have decisions to make. Each of the decisions you make will have an impact on your life, as well as the lives of the people who are close to you, including your family, your boyfriend, and your boyfriend's family. This is a big decision which needs to be carefully thought through. As you get started with this process, here are some things to think about:

- Feel good about yourself. Take a moment to think about all the things in your life which you have accomplished. Start a journal today. For your first entry write down all your good points.
- Maintain a positive attitude. Things have a way of turning out better when you think positively.
- Confide in someone you trust. Don't make your decision alone.
- Embrace the decision-making process. Be an active decision maker.
- Keep your mind open to all your options.
- Be determined. Recognize that your goal is to make the best possible decision for yourself and to get the appropriate care you need, no matter what you choose to do.
- Do something daily to boost your self-esteem. Take some time each day for yourself, whether it's to exercise or read a favorite book or magazine. Do something each day to help you feel good about yourself.

To Whom Can I Talk?

Sara wasn't able to concentrate in school all week. She received her algebra exam and found out she flunked it. Algebra was one of her favorite classes and Sara couldn't believe she had done so poorly. She felt bad about it. She cried even more. She didn't go to cheerleading practice all week. Her friends began bugging her, asking her lots of questions. She got in a fight with her best friend over something stupid. Sara didn't want to talk to anyone yet. It was Friday afternoon and Sara thought if she could just somehow get through the day, everything would be fine. Her English teacher caught her daydreaming in class and asked Sara a question. Sara was embarrassed because this was one of her favorite teachers. She had to admit she hadn't been paying attention at all during class. Sara was sure all her friends thought she was crazy. After class, her teacher asked to speak with her alone. Sara, feeling really upset, blurted out to her teacher that she was pregnant. Her teacher listened to her and encouraged Sara to talk to her mom. She gave Sara strategies on how to approach her mom, she even offered to help her. She put Sara at ease by telling her she wouldn't tell Sara's mom unless Sara asked her to. She gave Sara some

names and numbers of family planning clinics where she could get coun-
seling. Sara was surprised at how much better she felt after talking with
her teacher. She was relieved to talk to someone. She realized her teacher
cared about her.

It's important to talk to someone when you're faced with a difficult decision to make. As Sara found out, it can be very comforting to have someone you respect and who cares about you listen to your concerns. Sara was experiencing a difficult time and didn't know what to do. Sara took a risk, but by confiding in her teacher she got much-needed emotional support and appropriate guidance. Most important, Sara had been quite upset, and talking to her teacher made her feel tremendously relieved that she could rely on someone who cared about her.

It's not a good idea to make a decision alone. Involve as many trusted people you feel are necessary in order for you to make a clear decision. Your goal is to feel confident that you are making the best decision for yourself at this point in your life. When you are older, you want to be able to look back at this very important time in your life, and know that you did the best you could, that you made a well-thought-out decision. You don't want to look back and think to yourself, and say, "If only I had known . . . I would have . . ." For instance:

- If only I had known about open adoption
- If only I had known I could have had a second trimester abortion . . .
- If only I had known that if I raised my baby I would have to live with my mom . . .

Jennifer shares her experience in chapter 7. She was seventeen and a senior in high school when she got pregnant. She and her boyfriend married right away, but they separated six months after the birth of their daughter and were divorced a year later. This was a painful experience for Jennifer. She never thought about raising her child alone. Here's what Jennifer says:

I . . . felt trapped because I believed my only option was to get married and raise my child. It never occurred to me that I could raise my child alone. I was brought up to believe that it just wasn't done that way. . . . The divorce was very hard on me. It added another stressor for me on top of trying to be a good mother. Who knows if it would have been better for me to have stayed single and raised Emily on my own. Maybe I wouldn't have had to endure the abuse. Maybe I would have felt able to date sooner. Maybe I would have married sooner and had more children. These are things I'll never know.

Some young women don't think through all their options. They make their decision alone, or they do what someone else thinks they should do. Later on they wonder if they made the right decision. Courtney, who shares her experience in chapter 8, had an abortion when she was in college. She didn't consider all her options, she only talked to her boyfriend. She wonders today whether she made the best decision for herself. Courtney says, "As a result of not talking to anyone other than Steve, I never fully considered all my options. I made a decision at a time when I felt panic and fear, and I will always question whether my decision was sound and reasonable."

Joyce was fifteen when she became pregnant. Her mom and her boyfriend encouraged her to raise her baby. Joyce didn't consider any other options. At nineteen, she had just graduated from high school and didn't know what parenting involved when she became pregnant. Joyce says:

> Don't get me wrong, I love my daughter. She has brought a lot of joy into my life. There have also been some incredibly lonely and difficult times for me. I had no idea what I was getting myself into. Being a mother is hard work. It takes a lot of time, energy, and patience. Sure my mom helps, but my boyfriend's not around much. I never know whether I can count on him. I had our baby thinking he was going to help. He told me he was ready to be a father. The last four years have been tough. There are times when I'm exhausted. Sometimes I wish I had someone to take care of me. If only I had known how hard it would be without my boyfriend's help. I'm not sure, maybe I would have done things differently.

There are various options for you to consider, and you have to live with whatever option you choose. Only you know which option will work best for you in your situation.

Sara walked home from school, feeling a little better. She knew there was a lot ahead of her. She had to talk to her boyfriend, her mom, and her dad, but she felt a tremendous burden lifted. Suddenly there was a glimmer of hope. She felt she'd do okay. She decided to talk to her best friend first. She would have Jane come over after dinner that night. She would tell Jane then.

Sara's risk paid off. Her teacher gave her advice she needed and she felt more confident. She had already made one decision: She would speak with her best friend first. Confiding in someone is a risk. Once you disclose something sensitive about yourself, you can't take it back. You never know how the person will respond, and whether or not they'll keep your information private. This isn't meant to frighten you so that you don't confide in anyone. This is the risk you take when you reveal something about yourself. This is the risk you need to take if you're going to get the help you need. The trick is to balance your need for privacy with your need for support and information. Be selective about whom you share your pregnancy with. There are a lot of people who you can seek out for support and guidance. The following is a list of some of the people in whom you might confide:

- parent, guardian, aunt, uncle, godparent, or other responsible relative
- school nurse
- favorite teacher
- member of a religious group
- youth group leader
- family health care provider
- family planning counselor (for example, Planned Parenthood)
- mental health counselor

The individual in whom you confide should be someone you look up to, someone you respect, and someone you feel you can trust to maintain your confidence. Whoever you talk to should do the following things:

- be unbiased, nonjudgmental, objective
- help you feel comfortable expressing your feelings
- be someone who's interested in your success, who wants what's best for you
- be someone who can give you accurate information
- be someone who doesn't put down your feelings about your experience

Sara and Jane talked that night. Jane was shocked that Sara was pregnant. She said, "I can't believe you were so dumb." She was mad that Sara had been keeping the news from her. Jane offered her advice immediately: "Don't even bother to tell your boyfriend," she said. "Go get an abortion. I'll lend you the money if you need it. It's easy to get an abortion. Your mother doesn't ever have to know about it. It's the smart thing to do. You're fifteen, what do you want a baby for? Andy isn't going to hang around to

be a father," she warned her. "You made a mistake, now fix it, and get on
with your life." Sara was distressed by Jane's advice. She was counting on
Jane to listen to her. She wanted a shoulder to cry on. She was going to ask
Jane to go with her to the family planning clinic. Now she wasn't so sure
she wanted her around. Sara had never believed in abortion. She didn't feel
comfortable and was afraid she would get talked into something she didn't
want to do.

It's normal to want to talk to your friends first. It's probably easier for
you to talk to them. They probably know a lot about you already. Your
friends should help you, they shouldn't add to your problems, but your
friends may have inaccurate information. You need straightforward facts in
order to decide what's best for you. As Sara found out, friends may also try
to pressure you into doing what *they* feel is best for you. This may not be
what you want to do. Carolyn, who tells her story in chapter 9, told her best
friend about her adoption plans. Her friend was upset with her and was
against Carolyn's plan. Here's what Carolyn says:

I made the mistake of telling my best friend about my plans. She freaked
out. She started yelling at me, accusing me of being irresponsible. She told
me I would always regret my decision. She's my best friend. I was really
hurt by what she said. I thought she was open-minded and had liberal
views. Wow, was I shocked! I never anticipated how she would react. I was
counting on her to be more supportive of me.

Marie had a slightly different experience. Her best friend didn't agree
with her decision, but she offered her support anyway. Here's what Marie
says:

My best friend and I have been through everything together. I went to her
right away when I first found out I was pregnant. I know we don't always
agree with each other, but I can count on her to stand by me when I need
someone to lean on. I told her I was going to have an abortion. She told me
it was against her religious beliefs. She was sad that I felt I had to make
that choice. But she told me she would be supportive. She would still help
me out. She never passed judgment on me. She's a great friend.

You can't always know how someone will react. It's impossible to find
someone who's relatively unbiased. People are human. We all have our
biases. It's a good idea to prepare yourself that you may find someone who
doesn't react the way you want them to, or whose advice you don't like. You

may want to share your experience with more than one person. It may be helpful to have more than one viewpoint. Listen to what each person has to say, then make up your mind. Listen to your heart, and decide what's best for you.

Sara felt miserable the rest of the weekend. Her friends invited her to the movies, but she turned them down. She didn't feel like socializing. She called her boyfriend, Andy, on Sunday afternoon. He was upset by the news. Andy felt bad that she was pregnant. He acknowledged that he was also responsible. He offered to help her figure out what she was going to do. But, he told her he wasn't ready to be a father. He told her that he thought they should be dating others. He thought they were both too young for that kind of commitment. Sara started to cry. She really loved Andy. She was hoping that they would stay together. She thought he would stay in school, and she would live at her mom's house and raise their baby. Andy just kept saying that he wasn't ready to be a father. He also didn't want her to have an abortion, unless that was what she really wanted to do. They decided he would come home from college the next weekend so they could tell their parents together.

It was hard for Sara to hear that her boyfriend wasn't ready to be a father. She cried for a long time. Young men and women mature at different ages. Sometimes they have differing views about sex. Young men can view sex as something that's more casual, meant more for fun, and not necessarily romantic or leading to a commitment. Many young men don't want to be fathers or husbands at a young age. One study which interviewed teenage boys about their first sexual experience found that teenage boys were more likely than girls to view it as a casual experience. They were less likely to have feelings of commitment for their partner, and were also less likely than their partner to feel guilty about the sexual experience.[1] This had been Andy's first sexual experience. He had just started college. He was meeting other young women. He was being honest with Sara: He wasn't ready to be tied down. Even if your boyfriend doesn't want to be a father or husband yet, he's still partially responsible for your pregnancy. This is something that needs to be worked out between you and your boyfriend.

Sara's best friend, Jane, had a change of heart and told Sara at school on Monday that she'd had time to think about what Sara told her. She shared with Sara that she had had an abortion over the summer, so she knew what Sara was going through. Jane went through it alone; she was glad Sara had come to her for help. She told Sara she shouldn't have an abortion if it was against her beliefs. Sara and Jane went to a family planning clinic after school together where Sara had another pregnancy test. The clinician estimated that Sara was about nine weeks pregnant. She reviewed all of Sara's options and encouraged Sara to tell her mom. She told Sara she could bring her mom in. She offered to help Sara tell her mom. After the clinic visit, Sara and Jane had a long talk about abortion, and how Jane felt about her abortion. Sara was confused; having an abortion went against all of her beliefs. Yet Sara thought it might be best for her because she was young, and Andy wouldn't be involved raising the baby. She would be left raising a child on her own, and that she knew would be tough.

Sara realized she needed to tell her mom before the weekend. She had always gone to her mom before with her problems. Sara didn't want to bother her because her mother was upset about her own divorce, but now Sara felt she had to. The decision was getting too complex, and Sara felt overwhelmed. Sara wanted her mom on her side helping her. She wanted her mom's advice before Andy arrived.

The most important thing to do when you have a big decision to make is to collect information on all your options. Sara took a wise step: she collected valuable information. She found out how far along in her pregnancy she was, so she had an idea of how much time she had if she decided to terminate her pregnancy. Sara also began to explore her options. Sara had the chance to talk about abortion with a trained counselor, as well as with someone who had had one. It's important to remember that at this stage you're only collecting information. Going for abortion counseling doesn't mean you have to have an abortion. Going to see your health care provider doesn't mean you have to continue your pregnancy. Going for adoption counseling doesn't mean you have to place your baby for adoption. When you make these visits, you're collecting information that will help you clarify your decision. This will help you feel more confident that you've chosen the right option.

There are many options available to you for counseling. Many teens underestimate the value of talking to their current health care provider. Teens often categorize all adults as the same; they often conclude that their health care provider must be like their parents. They know their parents have opinions on drugs, sex, and cigarette smoking, so they think their health care provider does too. This is not so. Your health care provider has a much different role than your parents. Health care providers can give you clear, accurate information. If they've known you for a while then they have a good idea of your health history. It may be easier for you to talk to someone you know. They can guide you through the decision-making process. They can help you tell your parents. They can also refer you to community resources of which you may not be aware. Some teens are afraid that their health care provider won't maintain their confidentiality, but most health care providers have policies on confidentiality. They won't break that confidentiality unless your life is threatened. Angie talked to her doctor first. Here's what she had to say:

> I've had the same doctor since I was a little girl. I have asthma so I see her a lot. I've gotten to know her over the years. I trust her a lot. When I suspected I was pregnant I went to see her right away. My mom doesn't go with me to my doctor's appointments, so I was able to talk to her alone. I cried in her office when I found out I was pregnant. I didn't want to be. My mom is so strict. I didn't know how I was going to tell her. She helped me tell my mom. She helped us work out a plan.

TIPS FOR DEALING WITH YOUR HEALTH CARE PROVIDER

- Ask questions, be informed about the health risks to your body. Bring a list of questions with you to your appointment. Take notes if that helps you remember what was said.
- Be open and honest. Communicate all information that's necessary for your health care provider to know in order to treat you. Don't hide a bad habit if you have one, such as smoking cigarettes, drinking alcohol, or using illegal drugs. There are a lot of ways your health care provider can help you. There are educational videos you can watch, support groups you can attend, and special programs you can be referred to which can help you break your habit.
- Communicate your worries and fears. Try to be as clear as possible. Your health care provider can't read your mind.
- Don't avoid getting counseling or health care if you're concerned about your confidentiality being maintained. Every state has laws to protect an adolescent's confidentiality. Laws can vary from state to state. Ask your provider what his policy on confidentiality is.
- Make arrangements with your health care provider for communication of sensitive information. For instance, you can call your health care provider instead of having your provider contact you at home.
- If you're concerned about paying for health care, see if you can speak

to a social worker. A social worker may be able to find ways you can pay for your care. There may be a way you can be charged at a reduced rate. Also, you can pay in cash so a bill is not sent to your home.

* Remember, your health care provider was young once too. She knows the process may be difficult for you, that you may feel awkward about it. She is concerned about your health. She wants to make it as easy as possible for you.

Decision-Making Skills

Sara found out that making a major decision is difficult. There's a lot to consider. There's a lot at stake. You may also be feeling this way. Decision making is a skill. Most of us have never had a lesson on how to make a good decision. This is an important decision for you. Making a carefully thought-out decision will increase the chances that you will feel good about it. The decision process may seem overwhelming to you at times. You may get frustrated, angry, or sad, and this is normal. Everyone who's faced with a major decision experiences these feelings from time to time while they're making their decision. As you make this decision, you are laying down a foundation for the rest of your life for careful decision making. You are learning a valuable life skill. You are also more likely to make a better decision for yourself right now.

In any given day we make lots of decisions, perhaps as many as a dozen a day. Some of the decisions we make are minor decisions, like deciding what to wear to school or what to eat for lunch. Minor decisions are quick and simple to make. There's not much at risk, so we rarely think of the potential consequences.

There are other decisions we make in which there is more risk involved. Deciding to go to a party with your friends rather than study for a test is an example. There's bigger risk for you. There are also potential gains and losses for you. You'll probably have a lot of fun. You may meet someone new. This could be very exciting for you. However, if you fail your test, you may get a bad grade in that class. This may be a problem for you. Overall this decision may not have much of an impact on your life, but if you do this a lot there may be serious consequences. If you don't do well in school, you may not be able to go to the college or vocational school you want to. You may be disappointed in yourself. Your parents and teachers who know you are capable of doing better will also be disappointed in you.

Each decision you make has risks and consequences. Some decisions may be so small that you don't have to think about the potential risks or consequences. Others are major decisions. There are greater potential risks and consequences, both good and bad, which you need to consider. You have to live with your decision. Only you can decide the meaning of these consequences and whether the risk is worth taking.

The decision you are about to make is a major decision. It's a very important decision because it involves not only your life, but the life of your unborn baby and the lives of the people who are close to you. Here are some important aspects to decision making which may help you as you consider your alternatives.

Decisions have options. There are options available to you. You can choose to parent your baby, place your baby for adoption, or terminate your pregnancy. You can carefully decide which option is best for you, or you can let someone else make your decision. The choice is yours. You have to live with whatever happens. Only you can decide what's right for you to do.

Sometimes a young woman doesn't like her options and she doesn't want to make a decision. This happened to Gail. She spoke to a counselor, and was able to figure out what was bothering her. Here's what Gail had to say:

> All my options were bad options to me. I couldn't figure out how I was going to choose among what I considered three equally bad options. I felt helpless, which really bothered me. I like being in control. Finally my counselor helped me realize that I had a lot of anger. I was angry because I was pregnant, and that was something I couldn't change. I decided to be in control of my life. I thought through all my options and I chose the option which was best for me.

Decisions have consequences. Legally the decision how to handle your pregnancy is yours to make. However, each decision you make will have an impact on your life, as well as the lives of your parents or guardian, your family, your boyfriend, and his family. As you make this decision, you need to be aware of these possible consequences. If you're planning on raising your baby and you're going to live at home, you need to talk with your family about how your decision will have an impact on their lives. You need to work out a plan with your family. You need to respect how they feel.

Decisions have advantages and disadvantages. There is an advantage or gain, and a disadvantage or loss, associated with each option. What you lose, you can't get back. This is true for every decision you will make in your lifetime. For instance, if you decide you want to excel at playing the piano, you will have to practice a lot in order to accomplish this goal. You will experience a gain. You will have developed an artistic talent, something that you wanted to do very much. You will also experience a loss. You will have missed out on socializing with your friends and you may fall behind in your other activities. You can't get these missed opportunities back. No one can decide for you if this loss is so great that it wouldn't be worth the gain you would experience from being an expert pianist. This is a decision you have to make.

Similarly, there is an advantage and a disadvantage associated with each option that is available to you right now. You can read about these advantages and disadvantages in the chapters describing each option. As you consider each option, you need to carefully weigh the losses as well as the gains that you could experience with each alternative option. In that way you can decide which option is best for you. For instance, having an abortion is emotionally difficult, painful, and brings up a lot of feelings. Placing a baby for adoption is emotionally difficult, painful, and brings up a lot of feelings. Raising a baby is emotionally difficult, painful, and brings up a lot of feelings. No choice is pain free. You can't avoid loss, feelings of vulnerability, or painful emotions. However, there are advantages to each option. Make the time to carefully evaluate each advantage against each loss and determine which option is best for you.

Decisions relate to goals. The decision you make will have an impact on your short- and long-term goals. As you consider each option, think about how it will affect your life now, one year from now, and five years from now. Everyone has hopes, dreams, and desires about what he or she wants to accomplish during his or her life. The option that you choose will have an impact on your life now and throughout your life. Depending on the option you choose, you may have to postpone some of your short- and long-term goals.

Think seriously about your life and what you want. Take some time to identify both your short- and long-term goals. A short-term goal may be to save enough money to buy a bicycle or a CD player; or to graduate from high school. A goal for the near future may be to get accepted into college or vocational school. A long-term goal may be to graduate from college or vocational school, to have a career, to travel, or to develop a special talent. Your life will be affected by your decision. How your life goals will be affected is something only you can determine.

Decisions are based on values. Our values are our beliefs. They are the standards or codes which we live by. Our values are shaped by our families, friends, our religion, the media, and the society in which we live. Everyone's values are different. What you value may not be the same as what someone else values. You may value honesty, responsibility, loyalty, self-respect, family ties, education, having fun experiences, having freedom to do as you please, and so on. Adolescence is a time for discovering and refining your values.

Take some time to think about what your values are. Think about how your values may influence your decision. You may find that the option you choose is in conflict with your values. It doesn't mean you can't choose that option. It means you will have to find a way to resolve any conflict you are feeling.

Decisions require responsibility. You have the opportunity to set your own standards, to decide what is important to you based on what you feel is best for you. You have freedom to choose what is best for you. But with this freedom comes responsibility. If you decide to continue your pregnancy, whether you raise your baby or place your baby for adoption, you are responsible for keeping yourself physically healthy so that you and your unborn baby will be in good health. If you decide to terminate your pregnancy, you are responsible for keeping yourself physically healthy by getting a safe, legal abortion.

How Do I Know If I'll Be Satisfied with My Decision?

Sara wanted to talk to her mom. She thought about how she would approach her. She knew that when she spoke to her mom she did a lot better if she was clear about what her problem was, and if she could tell her mom some of the possible solutions. It was obvious to Sara what her problem was, but she wasn't sure what her solutions were. She didn't want an abortion; it went against her beliefs. She didn't think being a parent was a good idea either. She was confused about adoption. Sara was upset; she wasn't sure if any of the options were right for her. Sara wondered if she would ever be happy with any option she chose.

Sara had a valid concern. Whenever we make a decision we never know if we will be happy or satisfied with our choice. This is true for everyone who makes a decision. Taking responsibility for our decision and living with the consequences of it is something we all have to do. This is something that can be very scary. There are no guarantees that you'll be happy with your decision later. However, it's easier to accept a decision if you made it yourself than if it was forced on you.

There hasn't been much research to share with you that has looked at the level of regret or satisfaction with the decision process for abortion, childbearing, or adoption among teens, but a few studies have looked at the level of satisfaction among women who chose to terminate their pregnancies. This is what these studies found:

- Most women who have legal abortions in their first trimester of pregnancy do not experience serious psychological problems. Some studies have found that women who terminate an unwanted pregnancy feel their decision is psychologically better for them than carrying their baby to term.
- Women who feel they had more support for their abortion from their parents and boyfriend were more satisfied with their decision.
- Women who have fewer conflicts over abortion are also more satisfied with their decision.
- Women who had negative feelings toward their boyfriend, who made their decision alone, and whose parents were opposed to their decision to have an abortion experienced more emotional distress than those in opposite situations.[2]

You can't be certain that you will be satisfied with your decision. However, you can take steps to increase the likelihood that you will be satisfied with whatever you choose to do. Don't make a decision alone. Ideally you should discuss your decision with everyone who will be affected by whatever you choose to do. These studies suggest that family members play an important role in the decision-making process. It may not be possible for you to do that. Sometimes a young woman feels she can't talk to her parent or guardian or to the father of her baby. You will have to decide who you will involve with your decision process.

You may also have to make a decision which your parents or partner do not agree with. If this happens, try to get support from a trusted, caring adult. There are a lot of resources available to you. You should be able to find someone with whom you can discuss your decision. If you're making a decision which is in conflict with your beliefs, you may want to spend some time and sort out your feelings with someone who is objective. It's easier to sort these feelings out before you make a decision rather than after you make your decision.

Sara didn't sleep well that night. She was worried about telling her mom about her pregnancy. It took her a while to come up with a plan. As she left for school in the morning, Sara asked her mom if they could spend some time alone after dinner. Sara told her mom there was something bothering her that she wanted her advice on. Sara's mom agreed. She gave Sara a hug and told her she would speak with her later in the evening. Sara left for school dreading the upcoming conversation but knowing she needed to have it.

Most young women, like Sara, are nervous about telling their parents or guardian that they are pregnant. Sex is one of those sensitive issues which some teens don't feel comfortable talking about with their parents. Most teens assume a parent won't approve of premarital sex. It's normal for teens to struggle with their parents over values and lifestyle choices. This is part of growing up. The parents' basic instinct is to want to protect their child, while teenagers want independence and freedom to explore. Conflicts can and do arise which teens and their parents have to resolve.

If you've never talked to your parent or guardian about birth control or dating you may be even more worried about bringing up your pregnancy. Some pregnant teens tell their parents, usually their mother, but some pregnant teens choose not to tell their parents. You will have to decide whether you'll talk to your parents or guardian. You may want to consider that your parents or guardian may be angry at you and feel left out if you don't involve them with your decision process. Most teens do involve their parent or guardian with the decision-making process, and one study revealed that about 60 percent of all pregnant teens told one or both of their parents about their pregnancy even when they weren't required to by law.[3]

Before you talk to your parent or guardian it's a good idea to make a plan, like Sara did. Think about how you have dealt with decisions and conflicts in the past. Do you openly communicate with your parents or guardian when there is a problem which needs to be resolved, or do you make the decision alone and hope that they will agree with you? It's best to be open and direct with your parents. You may want to set aside some time to talk to your parents, like Sara did, when you can talk to them alone. It's probably best not to bring it up after they've had a bad day at work, or if they're in the middle of a crisis.

If you have trouble talking to your parents you may want to get the help of another adult. A relative, your health care provider, a family planning counselor, or teacher usually will be happy to help you. Your parent will probably be relieved knowing that you confided in a responsible adult.

You may want to start by telling your parents that you love them and value their advice. You may want to acknowledge to your parents that it's difficult for you to talk about what happened. Let them know that you're sorry that you've disappointed them. Be prepared that your parents may not be very happy. Most of the teens who shared their experiences say that their parents were shocked and angry with them, but once their parents got over their anger they helped the teens. Your parents may need time to calm down and deal with their own feelings before they're able to help you.

Alison, whose story is told in chapter 8, got pregnant when she was fourteen. Her parents had just finalized their divorce, and Alison was living with her dad. She didn't want to bother him because he was under so much stress at work and in his personal life. This is what Alison said:

> My dad had a lot going on at work, and he was working a lot of late-night hours. I didn't want to tell him at work, so I had to stay up late one night. I told him I was pregnant after he put in about a twelve-hour day at work. It wasn't exactly the best timing, but at that point I was desperate and had to tell someone. Once my dad got over his initial reaction he was fine.

⁂

Sara's mom was very upset about the pregnancy. She cried for a long time. She was angry at Sara. She let Sara know that she was disappointed in her. She had thought Sara had better judgment. Sara and her mom discussed her options. Her mom was also opposed to abortion, and she supported Sara's decision not to have one. Sara's mom had had high hopes for Sara. She had always assumed that Sara would go to college and establish a career before starting a family. Now that Sara's mother was getting a divorce, she was concerned about family finances. She didn't know how she would have the time or money to help Sara raise a baby. Sara had a lot of doubts about raising her baby. She didn't think she was in a position to be a good mother and provide adequately for her baby. She wasn't sure about adoption. She was worried that she might regret her decision later. Sara and her mom made a plan. Sara would start getting prenatal care and begin to explore both adoption and parenting her baby. Her mom agreed to go with her to see an adoption specialist, as well as to speak with her school about continuing her education and arranging day care if Sara decided to raise her baby. Sara planned to spend some time at a day-care center after school to see if she liked caring for babies. Even though her mom was upset, Sara was relieved to have confided in her, and to have her support. Sara's mom agreed to be supportive of her decision no matter what she chose to do, and to meet with Andy and his parents.

Sara had her mom's support. Even though her mom was not happy with her pregnancy, she agreed to help and be supportive of Sara. It's good to have your parent or another adult on your side. They can support you and help you sort out your feelings. Sara decided to continue her pregnancy, although she hadn't decided yet whether she would raise her baby or place it for adoption. Sara would have to carefully consider these options. She had a list of the people to whom she intended to speak.

THINGS TO CONSIDER

- Gather information and facts about each option. Speak to as many people as you can.
- Make a list of the pros and cons of each option.
- Carefully consider the pros and cons of each option, and how it will affect your life now and in the future.
- Be honest with yourself. You are making a decision which will have a lasting impact on your life, your family's life, your boyfriend's life, and his family's life.
- Gather more information if you need to. Reassess the pros and cons of each option before you make your final decision.
- Take an occasional break. The decision can be a difficult one to make. At times you may feel emotionally drained. By giving yourself an occasional rest you will have more energy and be better able to think clearly about what you want to do.

Sara's parents met with Sara, Andy, and his parents. It was an emotional gathering. Sara was glad she had her mom on her side. Andy's parents thought it would be best for Sara to have an abortion. They thought Andy and Sara were too young to be raising children. They were angry that Sara wouldn't consider an abortion. Reluctantly Andy agreed to help Sara financially if she chose to raise her baby, but he hadn't changed his mind. He wasn't ready to settle down yet. He didn't want to be a father, and he thought adoption was a better option for Sara. Sara was confused about her feelings. She was sad that she and Andy weren't continuing their relationship. She hadn't decided whether she would raise her baby or place her baby for adoption; she needed more time to make up her mind. Sara was going to meet with some teen moms, as well as continue to explore adoption. The adoption agency arranged for her to meet with other teens who had placed their babies for adoption, as well as an adoptive family.

This is an important decision. Gather all the facts you need to make your decision. Don't make a hasty decision. Carefully consider each option you have. Don't feel pressured to do what someone else thinks you should do. It's still your decision to make, even though your decision will have an impact on others. Sara had the support of her mother. She was going to continue her pregnancy, and at the same time carefully consider whether she would raise her baby or place it for adoption.

Some young women do not have the support of their families. This happened to Yolanda. She was seventeen and a junior in high school when she got pregnant. She very much wanted to raise her baby. Yolanda has made arrangements to live with an aunt, where she will be able to continue school and raise her baby. Yolanda explains:

> My mom and I haven't gotten along for a long time. We just don't see eye to eye on anything. She wants me to have an abortion. She wants me to graduate from high school and go on to college. She's afraid that I'm making the same mistake that she did. I know she loves her kids. She thinks my life is doomed if I have a child now. I know I'm smart. I love kids. It is part of my life's dream to have a baby. I tell her I'll go to college part-time. She says I won't be able to afford to and I'll be too tired. She doesn't want to be in a position where she has to help me. It's too painful for her. I can't live with her. She told me that if I want to be a parent, I'm on my own. I'm devastated. But I'm not letting her push me into an abortion. I'm lucky. My aunt has agreed to let me live with her. I'll have to get a part-time job, and help with the expenses. That's okay. I think that's fair. I know my life will be more difficult by having a child now, but this is what I want to do. I'm ready. I feel I can do it with my aunt's help.

Recap

The decision you are about to make can be overwhelming and complex. Don't make a hasty decision. Take the time to think through all your options. Take control of the decision-making process and make the decision which is best for you. Today there are many supportive services available. As Yolanda discovered, if you look you can find the resources you need. *You are capable of making this decision. You know what's best for yourself.* No one knows your life situation, your dreams, your desires, or what you want out of life better than you do yourself.

Take time to reflect on how your decision will impact on your life. Be calm when you're thinking about your decisions. Go somewhere by yourself. Take a walk in the woods or go to the beach. Listen to soft music. Think about your life. As you're thinking through your decision keep in mind these questions:

- What is to be gained if I choose this option?
- What is at risk for me?
- How will I feel if I don't choose this option?
- What will I need to carry through with my decision?
- Who are the people who can help me?
- What resources will I need, and how will I get them?
- How will this option affect my life now, one year from now, and five years from now?
- How does this decision impact on my life's dream? Where am I going? What do I want to accomplish?

Notes

1. K. D. Weddle, P. C. McKenry, and G. K. Leigh, "Adolescent Sexual Behavior: Trends and Issues in Research," *Journal of Adolescent Research* 3, nos. 3 and 4 (1988): 245–57 as cited in J. J. Card and S. Nelson-Kilger, *Just the Facts: What Science Has Found Out about Teenage Sexuality and Pregnancy in the U.S.* (Los Altos, Calif.: Sociometrics Corp., 1994), 16.

2. The research studies are summarized in the following two articles: N. E. Adler et al., "Psychological Responses after Abortion," *Science* 248 (1990): 41–44, and L. S. Zabin and V. Sedivy, "Abortion among Adolescents: Research Findings and the Current Debate," *Journal of School Health* 62, no. 7 (1992): 319–24.

3. S. K. Henshaw and K. Kost, "Parental Involvement in Minors' Abortion Decisions," *Family Planning Perspectives* 24, no. 5 (1992): 196–207, 213.

4

Becoming a Parent

It takes a whole village to raise a child.

African proverb

If you choose to parent your child you have a tough job ahead of you. Child rearing is a challenge no matter how old you are. There are personal gains and losses when you raise a child. It can be tremendously rewarding watching your child grow and thrive in life. Seeing life through the eyes of a young toddler as she experiments and discovers new things like going to the beach or playing in the snow for the first time can be very exciting. It can also be very frustrating trying to find the time and energy to care for your child, as well as to take care of your own needs. Chances are your life isn't settled yet. You're probably still in school, which means that more than likely you don't have a job and must rely on a parent or guardian for food, housing, and clothing.

A baby requires twenty-four-hour-a-day attention in a loving and stable environment with proper stimulation in order to grow into a healthy child. A baby's needs change as he grows. Choosing to be a parent means a commitment on your part for at least the next eighteen years of your child's life. Parenting is an enormous responsibility at any age. It's particularly more demanding now at this stage in your life because a baby demands so much of your attention at a time when you're growing from a teenager into an adult. It can be very frustrating trying to juggle going to school, maintaining friendships, and developing your own identity while caring for your baby.

It's not impossible for you to raise your baby. Should you choose to raise your baby, you will not be alone. Other teens before you have raised their babies. Of the one million teens who become pregnant each year, half (500,000) choose to raise their babies. All of those teens have discovered, however, that raising a child at a young age involves a lot of hard work. Parenting is an awesome responsibility that requires a total commitment on your part to work very hard to provide for both you and your baby. As a mother, you must place your child's needs before your own. You are always responsible for your child; however, you alone can't meet all your child's physical, emotional, and intellectual needs. You and your child need support. The stark reality about teen motherhood is that you will need a very strong support system in order to be a successful teen mom. This support system may take the form of a parent, a guardian, or another responsible adult or relative, help from the baby's father, and/or some type of specialized teen parenting program. Without additional help and resources the cards will be stacked against you. As the African proverb so aptly says, "It takes a whole village to raise a child." You can't do it alone.

Parenting has its advantages. Raising a child at a young age has given some teens an incentive to do better with their lives. Teen parenting has been a turning point in some young women's lives. They changed their old ways and lifestyles and in so doing improved their health as well as their baby's health. The quality of their life and their baby's life became that much better. Knowing they are responsible for a child makes them more determined to accomplish their goals. Their life takes on a new meaning. They learn very quickly about what's important to them. They recognize that they are responsible for themselves and their baby. Their number one goal is to be independent. Bringing a life into this world is an experience unique to a woman. Nurturing a life and watching a child grow, develop, and succeed can be very gratifying. Parenting can be a very positive experience for a young teen who's emotionally ready, and who has a very strong support system in place.

Parenting has its disadvantages. The responsibility of being a parent at a young age, especially if you are single, can be overwhelming. It's hard work raising a child, perhaps the toughest job that you will ever have. Many teen mothers are unable to get the kind of education that is needed today to get a good job. Because they have less education they end up working for low pay in service-type jobs such as staffing fast food restaurants, car washes, or as a housekeeper. The majority of teen mothers experience financial difficulties. With less pay they rely on their families or on public assistance payments for financial support at some point during their child's first five years of life. Having a baby will drastically change your lifestyle. This financial hardship will have a big impact on the quality of your life and your baby's life. Teen mothers are more likely to live in poverty during their teen and adult years than their peers who delayed having children until their late twenties or older. You may not be able to provide for your child the way you would like to, or the way that you were brought up. In addition, you may not be able to have the kind of lifestyle you would like for yourself. You won't have extra money to treat yourself to movies, makeup, or the latest clothing fashions.

When you choose to be a mother you are choosing an enormous responsibility. Your baby's needs will take priority over your own. Sacrifices will need to be made. This can be frustrating for you. It's unlikely that you will maintain the same friendships that you had before you were pregnant. There isn't time when you're juggling school, the baby, and possibly work. Teen moms want to be good mothers. They want to do a good job. Without an adequate support system it's very difficult if not impossible to do a good job. It can be very damaging to a young woman's self-esteem if she finds parenting more difficult than she expected or can handle.

What Choices Do I Have?

If you have made the decision to raise your baby, you still have choices: You can get married or you can stay single and raise your baby on your own, with or without the support of your baby's father. In the 1950s, when a young woman became pregnant she almost always placed her baby for adoption or she married the baby's father. Back then that was the way things were done. The young man did what was considered honorable. He married the woman he had gotten pregnant. Marriage was considered the "right thing" to do. Times have gradually changed. Abortion became legal in 1973, but even before that societal attitudes about sex outside marriage and single parenthood began to change. Now women have more options. Gradually over the years, more young women have chosen to either terminate their pregnancies or remain single and raise their child. Sometimes they get financial and/or emotional support from the baby's father, and sometimes they don't. If they don't get support, they raise their baby on their own. According to the Alan Guttmacher Institute, there has been a dramatic increase in the number of teens who are having their first baby outside of marriage. In the early 1960s, only 33 percent of first-time mothers remained single, whereas today 81 percent are choosing to do so. That's certainly a big change from earlier years. Unfortunately, staying single has the drawback of raising a child on one income, which is very difficult to do. Today, unmarried mothers and their children are more likely to live in poverty. Even when teen mothers become financially independent their lifetime earnings are only about half of what their peers who delay childbearing until their mid-twenties or older earn.

SHOULD I MARRY?

Marriage may seem like a good idea to you. Perhaps you and the baby's father have been in a long term relationship and are looking forward to marriage and the birth of your child. You may feel more comfortable raising a child at a young age if you're married.

Marriage has its benefits. If your relationship is strong you will have someone on whom you can rely to share child care responsibilities. It can be emotionally rewarding for you to share the highs and lows of parenting with the baby's father. It is also likely that you will be more financially secure. In today's economy it often takes two incomes to raise a family. It has been shown that married teens are much less likely to receive public assistance than teen moms who don't marry. However, your financial stability may last only as long as your marriage lasts. Many teen marriages are short-lived. Before you rush into marriage here are some important facts of which you should be aware:

- *Over one-half of teen marriages fail.* One study found that over half of teen marriages ended within five years, and for the women who stayed married, many complained of serious marital problems.[1]
- *Married teens often do not feel their spouse is emotionally supportive.* When researchers asked married teens to identify the two sources which they felt gave them the most emotional support, surprisingly, only one in three of the married teens identified their spouse as a source of emotional support.[2]
- *Married teen mothers are at high risk of having a second birth within two years of the first birth.* A second baby places even more strain on their marital relationship.[3]

The statistics look grim. Teen marriages may very well start out with all good intentions, but they tend to be unstable. If you're considering marriage now, you might want to consider how you would feel if your marriage ended in divorce. Raising a child at a very young age is difficult enough; experiencing a divorce or marital woes may make it that much more difficult for you to raise your child. Teen moms who marry tend to have another baby soon after the first. If they divorce they are left with considerable financial hardship. Raising two children on one salary can be very difficult. Child support payments from teen dads tend to be small because teen dads have lower salaries and so their ability to provide financial support is poor.

In chapter 7, you'll read about Jennifer, who was a senior in high school when she became pregnant. She and her boyfriend, Tom, married when she found out she was pregnant. Tom had just graduated from college and had a good job, but their marriage didn't last long. Jennifer's idea of married life was different than Tom's. Jennifer had expected that Tom would help out more with child care, for example. Tom just wasn't ready for marriage. He complained of feeling "trapped" and became abusive. Within six months of their marriage Tom and Jennifer separated and they divorced a year later. Jennifer and her baby had to move in with her parents for a while. Jennifer experienced financial difficulties for a long time, and she raised her daughter by herself.

Of course, not all teen marriages end in divorce. Some marriages are successful and beat the odds. Dan and Diane are an example of a successful teen marriage. They were married right out of high school when Diane got pregnant. They have been married for ten years now. With the help of their families, they made it through the rough times. What worked for them? Diane says:

> We're both too stubborn. We didn't want to be a statistic. We enjoy raising our son together. Sure it was a struggle. We had some tough times. Dan was just as committed to our marriage and to raising our son as I was. We switched child care around, so we could both go to school and work. We've been crazy about each other since we were kids. We have the same values. Both sets of our parents were also supportive and helped us out from time to time.

Getting married is a serious decision. For a marriage to be successful it requires a great deal of maturity, as well as a mutual commitment to each other and to the marriage. If you and your boyfriend are considering marriage you may want to talk to your parents, someone from your church, or counselor to see if you're both ready to take on the additional responsibility which marriage involves. There may also be legal aspects to consider, depending on which state you live in (for example, most states have minimum age requirements for a marriage to take place).

Decision-Making Process

Having a baby at a young age can have serious consequences for you and your baby, the baby's father, and your families. Choosing to be a mother is a big responsibility. Your life and the lives of the people close to you will be affected. This is a serious decision. Carefully considering these questions may help you determine if motherhood is right for you at this point in your life:

Do you have a realistic view of what your child's needs will be?
    Newborns need to be fed and diapered every two to three hours, around the clock. This is a twenty-four-hour-a-day job, every day of the year. In order to thrive babies need a loving, supportive environment with proper stimulation. As babies grow to be toddlers, they nap less, they're awake more. They ask lots of questions. They're discovering how the world works and they want you to teach them. They need even more of your attention. A child needs toys and a safe place to play. You may not get a break until your child enters the first grade. And even then your child will need help with homework, and car rides to and from school and activities like soccer practice, gymnastics, etc.
    Try out parenting. Babysit for someone's baby or toddler, or spend some time taking care of children in a day-care center. Remember that when it's your child no one will pay you, and you don't get to go home at the end of the day when you're tired. Your baby has needs. You have needs. Becoming a mother is a full-time commitment to care for your child. It can get frustrating if all your time and energy is devoted to your baby and you feel you don't have time for yourself.

What are your reasons for wanting to be a parent?
    Do you expect your child to make your life complete? Are you hoping that if you have this baby, you and your boyfriend will stay together, or that your parents will love you more or take you more seriously? The father of your baby may start out with good intentions, but may not remain involved. Parenting and being in a mutually committed relationship is not only a choice; it requires readiness. Some teen dads find out that they're not ready for that kind of commitment or responsibility. If you have your baby for

your boyfriend, how will you feel about your baby if your boyfriend is no longer involved with you or her? If you have your baby because your parent encourages you, how will you feel if your parent doesn't give you the kind of support you want or feel you need?

Are you trying to prove to your parents that you're mature, that you're an adult now?

Having a baby may place more stress on your relationship with your parents. Instead of becoming more independent, you will become dependent on your parents or another adult until you can support yourself and the baby on your own. Being dependent on an adult at this point in your life may be frustrating and uncomfortable for you.

Are you emotionally prepared to be a parent now?

Do you enjoy playing with children? How did you like babysitting? Were you patient? Did you get frustrated by the demands of the child? Were you looking forward to the end of the day when you could go home? Having a child requires an incredible amount of patience and you will not be able to go home at the end of the day and leave the baby, its demands, and your frustration behind.

How do you feel about yourself? Do you feel you're doing a good job in school? Are you confident in your ability to have a goal, make a plan, and carry it through until you've accomplished your goal? If you choose parenting, you have lots of goals ahead of you. You need to find day care so you can graduate from high school. You'll need to find a job so you can support both yourself and your baby.

Do you have the financial resources to raise a child?

Do you have a place to live? Have your parents agreed to let you live with them? Will you have to pay rent? Do you have health care insurance for both you and your baby? Will you be able to buy formula, diapers, and clothing for your child? Children grow quickly and can grow out of their clothing every few months. All these things can be very expensive.

Babies need more than love and care. Take out a paper and pencil, and figure out a monthly budget. Your budget should include the amount of money you think it will cost for food, formula, diapers, medicines, day care, babysitter costs, and emergency expenses. Figure out how much money you think you will be able to earn. Next go out and price everything. Did you have money left over? Did you run up short? If you want to go to a movie once a month, you'll need a babysitter. Does your budget allow for it? You'll need day care so you can continue with your schooling. Were you able to find day care at your school? Were you able to find day care at a price which you can afford? Now go out and price the baby's nursery. You'll need more than a crib. You'll also need baby sheets, baby blankets, a thermometer, a stroller, and a car seat. Sometimes you can get these things for a reasonable price at a second-hand store, or your friends may lend you something. Many single teen moms qualify for public assistance programs. But even being eligible for and receiving assistance will not solve all your financial problems. Most states are changing eligibility requirements, making it harder for some teens to get assistance. Tonya tell us: "It's a real struggle supporting my daughter on welfare. It's barely enough money to survive. I don't think anyone should rely on welfare. I always feel like everyone discriminates against you." Some moms can also qualify for Women and Infants and Children (WIC), which can provide coupons for nutritious, essential foods. These programs may help your finances, but they don't cover all the costs of parenting.

Do you have a support system in place?

You need a strong, supportive network of family, friends, and/or members of your faith on whom you can rely when you need help. It's also helpful to have one person who shares your goal of parenting. A strong support system is an absolute necessity in order for you to succeed at parenting. As one midwife explains, "I tell all my patients to identify someone right away who will be their pinch hitter, who will be at their side, who will go the race with them." You need someone who will be invested in you and in your success as a teen mom. This support person may not be your boyfriend. Parenting is a real challenge, and he may not be ready for it. It may not be one of your parents; they may not be able to take on this role. You might have to look to an aunt, a grandmother, or a godmother to help you. Remember, teens who make it have a very strong support system.

Changes Up Ahead

Raising a child at a young age can be very difficult. All new mothers feel pressures when they have a baby because a baby places a strain on a family's finances and relationships. These pressures can be even more difficult for teen mothers because there are so many areas in their lives which are not settled yet. You can expect some changes in your education, finances, and relationships with family and friends. Depending on your home life you may experience even more changes. If you're currently growing up in a home where you don't feel emotionally supported or you don't have enough money to get by, you may have an even more difficult time adjusting to parenting. Think about your home life now. Is there alcohol or drug abuse, violence, unemployment, lack of food or clothing, or inadequate housing? If you are in a bad home situation now, it will be that much harder for you to care and provide for a baby. The additional stress of caring for a child can further disrupt a home that's already having trouble. This may place you and your child at risk. This may not be what you want to read; it may be difficult for you to think about this, but assessing your home life and your support systems now may help you to plan ahead to find the resources which you will need. You may also decide that you're already experiencing a difficult time in your life and that this isn't the right time for you to have a baby.

EDUCATION

Teen moms have made some educational advances throughout the years. More teen moms are graduating today from high school than in the 1970s. This is because federal legislation was passed in the 1970s to protect the rights of teen students. It is illegal for schools that receive federal funds to expel students who are pregnant or are parents. *You cannot be expelled from school because you're pregnant or a teen parent.* Also, many schools are making it easier for teen mothers to go to school. Some schools have on-site day care, making it easier for teen mothers to attend classes. Other schools have alternative programs for pregnant teens, teen mothers, and their babies. Because these programs are run separately from the school, some pregnant teens and teen mothers feel more comfortable going to school and continuing their education.

The good news about education for teen mothers:

- A teen mom who has her baby while she's in school and who stays in school is just as likely to graduate as a teen who did not have a baby.[4]

The bad news about education for teen moms:

- Among high school dropouts, teens who have a baby are less likely to go back.[5]

- Teen moms are less likely to attend college than women who postpone childbearing.[6]

Education today is more important than ever. The prospects of getting a good job with a high school diploma or less are not very good. Less education means work requiring no special skills which means low pay. This is why so many teen moms struggle financially to support their baby. According to the United States Department of Commerce, the average monthly income in 1993 for persons between the ages of eighteen and twenty-four years old based on the highest level of education they had reached is as follows:

Not a high school graduate	$ 459/month
High school graduate only	$ 783/month
Some college, no degree	$ 610/month
Vocational training	$1,017/month
Associate's degree	$ 912/month
Bachelor's degree	$1,128/month
Master's degree	$1,351/month[7]

These figures show some tough facts. If you're a high school dropout there's no doubt that you will have a tough time supporting yourself and your baby. It's going to be hard to support yourself and a baby with only a high school diploma. A college degree or some type of vocational training will increase your chances of getting a better-paying job, which will make it easier for you to support yourself and your baby.

So you can see, it takes vocational training or a college degree today to get a good job with a good income. Many single women today know that they need more than a high school degree in order to support themselves and are delaying childbirth in order to get more education and to advance their careers. With so many college-educated women looking for jobs it makes it that much more difficult for a teen mother with little education to compete in the job market and get a job that pays well.

FINANCES

It's expensive to raise a baby. Many teen moms have limited finances and struggle to raise their babies. What makes it hard for them is that before they became pregnant many started out living in poverty or low-income homes. Many teen moms live with one parent, usually their mother. Oftentimes there isn't enough money to get by to begin with, and then a baby comes along and places a real burden on the family. The majority of teen moms do not marry the baby's father. They are left to support themselves with the help of their families, whatever limited income they might have, or they rely on welfare payments. Some teen moms have a second baby within two years of their first baby. One child places a strain on your finances; an additional child will make it that much harder for you to complete your education and find a job to support yourself and your children.

As Tonya explains:

> I don't think you can understand being poor unless you've lived it. I barely have enough money to get by. Sure, I receive medical assistance and welfare payments for myself and my baby, but it's never enough. I always feel like people discriminate against me because I'm on welfare. I try hard. I pay my bills. All my money goes to bills and for my baby. I can't do little things like treat myself to an ice cream sundae or buy earrings for myself. I haven't bought clothes for myself in ages. Plus, I don't have a car. I have to rely on public transportation. Sometimes I need to take three different buses to get to a doctor's appointment. When my baby's sick it's a real hassle. It hurts me that I have to put my baby through all that when she's not feeling well.

If you're thinking about having a baby now, this could also happen to you. You may not have adequate finances to raise your baby the way you want to. It can be very frustrating for you if you don't have enough money for the bare necessities for yourself and your baby.

The bad news about finances for teen moms:

- Teen moms are more likely to rely on public assistance to pay for prenatal care and to raise their child than older mothers.
- Teen moms are more likely to be poor during their teen and adult years than their peers who delay parenting until their twenties and older.
- Overall, teen moms make only half the family income of their peers who postpone childbearing until after their mid-twenties.[8]

The good news about finances for teen moms:

- Twenty years after the birth of their baby the majority of teen moms have finished high school, gotten stable jobs, and have become completely self-supporting. Some moms, however, continue to struggle and live in public housing.[9]

You can catch up. Teen parenting does not mean that you are doomed to a life of poverty. It will require a lot of hard work on your part. You may be willing to endure the short-term financial difficulties that other teen moms experience, knowing that if you work hard, in the long term you and your baby will overcome your initial hardship.

CHANGES IN YOUR RELATIONSHIPS

Having a baby places a strain on all the important relationships in a woman's life. This happens to any woman who has a baby; even older women who are in stable, married relationships experience some changes in their lives with the birth of a baby. They too must juggle their time and deal with changed roles with their spouses, family, and friends. Depending on your family, your home life, and your boyfriend, the changes in your relationships which you experience may make it more difficult for you. You are probably living in your parents' home, which makes you financially dependent on them. They might not be thrilled about having a baby in their home. They may not want the emotional or financial burden. Some parents respond with anger and distress when their unmarried daughter becomes pregnant. They may be angry at you for getting pregnant, as well as angry at your boyfriend for getting you pregnant. As Janna says:

> I got tired of the cold treatment my father kept giving me. He made it very clear he did not want me to have my baby. I couldn't take living at home while he was acting toward me in that way. I had a friend who had already graduated from high school and was living in her own apartment. I moved in with her. I got a part-time job to pay the rent. It's tough, but I only have six months of school left. It's better for my emotional health this way.

Janna experienced a change in her life. She no longer had the financial or emotional support of her parents. She experienced a tougher time, but in the end she was able to cope.

Sonya's story is a little different. Sonya had her baby, mostly because her boyfriend pressured her to. At first her parents were upset about her pregnancy, but now they are supportive. Her boyfriend was also supportive of her pregnancy, but has since changed his mind. Sonya is upset about this. She wanted his support. She's hoping that he will come around, but she knows at this point that he probably won't.

You may also experience changes with your peers. Some of your friends may not approve of your pregnancy. As Tricia says:

I don't think there's any less stigma today when you're single and raising a child on your own. When I walk down the halls at school, some of my friends walk the other way. It's like they definitely don't approve of my having a baby on my own. Still it would be nice to have their support.

No matter what choice you make, your friends and families may not approve. It's still *your* decision to make. These changes will probably cause you some distress. This is only normal. It helps to have some stability in your life, like the support of an older friend or a parent. It also helps to be able to talk about these feelings with someone you trust.

Of course the opposite can also happen. You may want to spend more time with your friends, and find it difficult to deal with the fact that you have less freedom. All these changes with the important relationships in your life can cause you stress and anxiety. It's important for you to know that these changes may occur, so that you can take steps to deal with them. Being around people who are supportive will help you cope better during your pregnancy and when you parent. If the people around you aren't supportive you can reach out to members of your faith and your community.

Am I Doomed for Life?

You are *not* doomed for life. The statistics you've read reflect trends in teen parenting. You don't have to be a statistic. If you work hard and get the resources you need, you can live a fulfilling life. You and your baby don't have to live a life of poverty and isolation. Teen mothers who have succeeded have done so because of personal drive, inner strength, and a willingness to change so that they and their baby's lives could be better. Over and over we hear teens say, "I don't want to be a statistic." Teens want to do a good job at parenting. In chapter 7, you'll read Jennifer's story. Her marriage ended within a year of her child's birth. She made sacrifices and changes in her life for the sake of her baby. When her marriage ended, she moved into her parents' home until she was financially independent. She took a job in a factory. She only had a high school diploma, and the job didn't pay much. It was what she considered menial work, which didn't give her any personal satisfaction, but it gave her the best pay she could find, health insurance for her and her baby, and a work schedule which allowed her to stay at home during the day with her baby. She worked part-time and went to college. With scholarships, day care, and support from her parents she was able to graduate. She has a stable job now and owns her own home.

Her child is in high school and is at the top of her class and has plans to go to medical school.

Dianne Wilkerson shares another personal success story on teenage pregnancy. When Dianne became pregnant in high school, she faced some of the same obstacles other pregnant teens face, telling her mother, continuing her education, and creating goals for herself and following through with them. Today Dianne is a mother, as well as a lawyer, and the first African-American female state senator in Massachusetts. Dianne says:

> I didn't know that I wanted to be a lawyer or a politician when I was young. All I knew was that I enjoyed learning. I knew that I had to stay in school so that I could be in the best position to take care of my baby. I owe my success to my family. I was able to accomplish my goals because my family was behind me. They knew I needed to stay in school, so they pitched in and shared child-care responsibilities. I was able to go to school and know that my baby was well cared for.

Dianne offers this advice to other pregnant teens:

> Feel good about yourself, feel good about your life and your goals. Don't give up on yourself. Your life is not over because you are pregnant. Your baby will be the most important part of your life. Child rearing is not easy. It's difficult, but it's not impossible. There may be obstacles and bumps along the way which may make you angry and frustrated. If you put your mind to it, you will succeed. Stay in school. Your education is an investment in yourself. Every investment you make in yourself is an investment in your baby. There are many resources available to help you. Ask for help if you need it. When people see that you want to achieve they will help you.

How to Succeed

Below are four steps which you can take to become a successful teen mother. These are steps other teen moms have taken which have helped them overcome the burden of early child rearing.

1. Get good prenatal care. Many research studies have demonstrated that early and consistent prenatal care increases the likelihood that a teen mom will deliver a healthy baby. According to the Guttmacher Institute, one-third of pregnant teens receive inadequate health care. Many teens are afraid to tell their families they are pregnant, they lack health insurance, they're afraid to go to a health care provider, or they don't realize prenatal care is important. Getting early and regular prenatal care is important for your health and your baby's health. Your health care provider will monitor your health closely and be able to pick up problems right away, which will increase your chances of delivering a healthy baby.

Lifestyle changes are also key. Maintaining a healthy lifestyle is a good idea whether you're pregnant or not. When you're healthy you feel better about yourself and you enjoy life more. The added demands that a growing baby places on your body requires that you take extra good care of yourself now. Eating well-balanced, nutritious meals, getting the right amount of rest and exercise, as well as reducing stress in your life will be good for both you and your baby. If you're struggling with some unhealthy habits like drinking alcohol, using illegal drugs, or smoking cigarettes, let your health care provider know. There are special programs to which she can refer you to help you quit or start cutting back on any of these habits. Changing these habits is a way you can do something good for yourself and your baby. You'll feel a lot better about yourself too.

Teens who followed a special prenatal care program were found to be less likely to deliver an underweight baby (less than five and a half pounds, also called low-birthweight) than those who did not follow such a program.[10] The best prenatal care program is one which offers nutrition counseling as well as social service support in addition to obstetrical care. A social worker is not someone of whom to be afraid. She can help you find day care, enroll you in childbirth and parenting classes, provide you with emotional support, and help you to find a way to stay in school. Most communities have these programs. Your school nurse can help you find one, or you can look in the Yellow Pages under "Pregnancy." Remember, if your baby is healthy it will be that much easier for you to take care of him.

2. *Continue with your education.* In order to get a well-paying job today, you need your education. If possible, take advantage of on-site day-care programs at your school. Day care can be expensive. A social worker connected with your school or prenatal care provider may be able to help you locate good but inexpensive day care. A family member may be willing to babysit. Teens who have day care are more likely to stay in school and graduate. Teens who drop out of school frequently do not return to graduate. One thing to keep in mind is that if you're already doing poorly in school, having a baby will only make it harder for you. You may be tired from being up all night, which could make it harder to concentrate in class. Also, because of the baby, you may not have time to study as much, which may make it more difficult for you to graduate.

3. Gather a strong support system. It takes lots of support to be a good teen mom. Teens who have a strong support system that includes family, friends, church, and community do a better job with parenting. The ability to parent is not a biologically inherited trait. Because you are a woman does not mean that you will automatically know how to parent. You'll need lots of people to whom you can turn for guidance with child care and for emotional support. Try to find one person who's interested in your success, who will go the extra mile for you. This is important because you never know when you may need help. For instance, if you don't have a car, you'll need someone who is willing to take you to the emergency room in the middle of the night if your baby's very sick.

A strong, supportive, home environment is also important. Teen moms who receive child-care assistance from another adult feel more comfortable in their role as a mother and are more competent with parenting skills than are teens who raise their child alone. Teens are also more likely to stay in school after they have their baby if they live at home with their parents. If they move out they are more likely to drop out of school. Evita explains:

> I was scared, nervous, and needed lots of help caring for my daughter. My mom was there for me. I was lucky to have someone that stood by me. My advice for other pregnant teens is to have someone there to help you. Also, take care of your own needs, finish high school, and have goals. Above all, always believe in yourself.

4. Space Your Pregnancies. About 30 percent of teens who have their first child before they are seventeen and about 25 percent of those who are under eighteen or nineteen will have another baby within two years of their first baby.[11] Teen mothers who marry are also more likely to have closely spaced births.[12] These teen mothers have a more difficult time staying in school. They also receive less prenatal care, and they tend to have sicker babies at birth. Once you have two children, your life will become that much more complicated. It may be more difficult for you to get to school, as well as to your prenatal appointments and to the baby appointments.

THINGS TO CONSIDER

If you're planning on raising your baby, it's a good idea to start thinking about the future. This will help you prepare for yourself and your baby. Answering these questions is a good starting point. Discuss these questions with your family, your guardian, and/or your boyfriend. You'll be able to make a better plan if you're open and honest with the people who will be helping you with your baby. As with any plan, things can change, so it's also good to have a back-up plan in place.

- Where will you live while you're pregnant and after your baby's born?
- How will you continue school? Do you have day care arranged for your baby? Do you have transportation from your home to your school?
- Who's your number one support person that you can count on if you need help?
- Who are your back-up supports? Are there friends, relatives, or church members that can help you from time to time? If so, how much support can you expect from them?
- Will the father of your baby be involved? How will he help? Can his parents help?
- Do you have health insurance for yourself and for your baby?
- What personal goal(s) do you want to accomplish this year?
- Where do you want to be five years from now?
- What steps do you need to take over the next five years to accomplish this goal?

Effects on Your Baby

A baby born to a teen mother can have more health problems than a baby born to an older mother. Teen mothers deliver more babies who are underweight at birth (under five and a half pounds, also called low-birthweight) compared to other mothers. Oftentimes these babies are born too early and their organs are not fully developed. They can suffer serious lung problems or experience bleeding in their brains. These babies are much more likely to die in the first month of life than normal weight babies. Some underweight babies that live do fine. Other underweight babies experience many medical and developmental complications throughout life. Maintaining a healthy lifestyle while you're pregnant and getting early and regular prenatal care can increase your chances of delivering a healthy, full-term baby.

Babies born to teen mothers tend to experience developmental delays more often than babies born to older mothers. This can happen even when your baby's weight is normal at birth. These developmental delays can begin when the baby is young and may continue throughout the child's school years. This means that these children may take a longer time than normal to learn some skills (such as walking and talking). Preschool children of teen mothers have been found to be more active, more aggressive, and to have less self-control than children of older mothers. Older children of teen mothers don't do as well in school, and they score lower on standardized intellectual achievement tests. They are more likely to fail a grade in school. Children who are aggressive in school don't learn as well and they also don't fit in. This makes it harder for them to develop friendships, because other children are afraid of the aggressive behaviors.

Some of the reasons why children of teen mothers don't do as well are that they tend to grow up in poverty, unsafe neighborhoods, and home environments which aren't very stable. It may also be related to the parenting skills of teenage parents. Some teen mothers may not respond appropriately to their children. This is not because they don't want to, it's because they don't know how to. They are unable to nurture their child because they were never nurtured as children, or because they're emotionally exhausted from the pressures of their lives. It's important to keep in mind that not all babies born to teen mothers will experience developmental delays and do poorly in school. Just as you are not doomed if you choose motherhood at this time in your life, your baby does not have to be doomed either. Taking a parenting class may help you feel more comfortable with child development and appropriate activities you can do with your child. Also, having positive role models around to assist and support you will help.

Loss Associated with Parenting

Each teen's reasons for choosing parenting are different. Some teens become parents because they think it is the responsible thing to do. Some do so because they want to be parents. Some choose parenting because they think the emotional pain associated with adoption and abortion would be too great. These teens think that by choosing parenting, they can escape the feelings of grief or loss which they would experience if they chose another option. You will experience a loss no matter which option you choose. There are losses associated with raising your child which will cause you some grief and pain. How much the losses will affect you depends on the supports and resources you have as well as your personality type. Below are some of the losses which you may experience.

Your Childhood. You will have less time and energy to discover who you are, what you like to do, and what you want to do with the rest of your life. You will become the nurturer, that is, you *give* endless care instead of receiving it. Most teenagers are trying to become independent from their parents. Having a baby now will make you more dependent on your parents and for a longer time than if you didn't have a baby. Having fun is an important part of adolescence. It may be hard for you to cut back on your social life.

Your Education. It may be difficult for you to pursue an education because of financial reasons as well as lack of time. If you're already having a difficult time in school, having a baby will only make it that much more difficult for you to complete your education. As Karen puts it:

> My baby would be up all night, sick with an ear infection or just cranky. It didn't matter that I had been up all night, I still had to get up and get to school. If my baby was sick and couldn't go to day care, I had to find someone else to care for her. It's a constant struggle. I feel I never have enough time for myself and I'm always rushing with my baby. I don't have time to really enjoy her.

Your Social Life. You will have less time and energy to spend with your friends. If you do go out you need to get a babysitter, and you need to have the extra cash to pay for one. Your priorities and your interests will change. Sometimes it will be difficult for you to find friends that are interested in both you and baby, and are willing to be flexible enough to accommodate your schedule. Let's face it, most young people don't want a young child around when they're out having a good time.

Your Privacy. This is a day-to-day loss which you will experience. Your baby and especially your toddler will always be with you. You will have little time to do any of the following things alone: take a shower, put on your makeup, go to the bathroom, talk on the phone, go shopping, eat a peaceful meal, read a magazine, or even sleep. Basically, everything you do revolves around your baby's needs and schedule. For example, you may be trying to get to school on time, but your toddler will interfere with your schedule. That's because your toddler will want your attention and will need to be fed, washed, and dressed.

SUGGESTIONS FOR COPING WITH PARENTING

- Involve your boyfriend and family or another adult with your decision making. Identify at least one person who will be there for you. Have a clear understanding from them as to what they will be capable of doing to help you out.

- Explore all your financial resources. Most parents' health insurance policies will cover the cost of your prenatal care and possibly your baby's care. Ask your parents to check with their employer. There may be special restrictions. For instance, you may be required to be a full-time student in order to receive health care coverage. If you can't get assistance from your parents, you may be eligible for public assistance. Your local welfare office can assist you through the application process and help you enroll in other programs for which you might be eligible, such as WIC.

- Keep focused on your education and personal goals.

- Many schools have special programs which will allow you to continue your education while you're pregnant and when you're raising your baby. Home tutoring can usually be arranged if you need to stay at home. Some schools have day care on site, or can help you arrange day care. There are also alternative schools for pregnant and parenting teens which you can go to. You may feel more comfortable studying only with students who are pregnant or parenting. Your guidance counselor can assist you with the right school program.

- Don't be afraid to ask for help. Let your boyfriend, parents, and friends know when you need a break. There are other resources available if your friends and family can't help. Most communities have teen parent programs. You can look in the Yellow Pages under "Pregnancy" for a list of these programs.

- Spend your free time with achievers. There are other teens who are working very hard to succeed at parenting. Form your own supportive networks. It's always better to be a part of the "I can" crowd rather than the "misery loves company" crowd.

- Use reliable contraception to space future pregnancies. Having another child right away will only complicate your life. Financially and emotionally it will be much harder for you to care for your children as well as complete your education.

- Be good to yourself. Take good care of your physical and emotional health. By eating right, getting exercise and proper rest you will have more energy to care for your child and accomplish your goals. Talk to a close friend about your feelings. Joining a support group of young teen parents can also help you understand that what you are experiencing is normal.

Notes

1. J. J. Card and S. Nelson-Kilger, *Just the Facts: What Science Has Found Out about Teenage Sexuality and Pregnancy in the U.S.* (Los Altos, Calif.: Sociometrics Corp., 1994), p. 72.

2. Ibid.

3. F. L. Mott, "The Pace of Repeated Childbearing among Young American Mothers," *Family Planning Perspectives* 18, no. 1 (1986): 5–12.

4. D. M. Upchurch and J. McCarthy, "The Timing of a First Birth and High School Completion," *American Sociological Review* 55 (1990): 224–34.

5. Ibid.

6. The Alan Guttmacher Institute, *Sex and America's Teenagers* (New York: Alan Guttmacher Institute, 1994), p. 60.

7. "Mean Monthly Income by Highest Degree Earned: 1993," *Statistical Abstract of the United States 1995*, 115th ed. (Washington, D.C.: United States Department of Commerce).

8. The Alan Guttmacher Institute, "Teenage Reproductive Health in the United States," *Facts in Brief* (pamphlet), August 31, 1994.

9. S. M. Horowitz et al., "School-Age Mothers: Predictors of Long-Term Educational and Economic Outcomes," *Pediatrics* 87, no. 6 (1991): 862–68.

10. D. M. Carter et al., "When Children Have Children: The Teen Pregnancy Predicament," *American Journal of Preventive Medicine* 10, no. 2 (1994): 108–13.

11. Guttmacher Institute, "Teenage Reproductive Health."

12. Mott, "The Pace of Repeated Childbearing."

5

Is Abortion the Right Choice for Me?

Reproductive freedom—the fundamental right of every individual to decide freely and responsibly when and whether to have a child—is a reaffirmation of the principle of individual liberty cherished by most people worldwide. It helps ensure that children will be wanted and loved, that families will be strong and secure, and that choice rather than chance will guide the future of humanity.

Planned Parenthood Federation of America Mission Statement

Abortion is one option which is available to you. Today all women in this country have the legal right to an abortion. That has not always been the case. For many years abortion was illegal in the United States. Even when abortions were illegal many women risked their lives and health in order to terminate an unwanted pregnancy. An Institute of Medicine report estimates that as many as one million illegal abortions were performed each year prior to the legalization of abortion.[1] Interestingly, that figure is close to the number of legal abortions which now occur each year in our country. According to the Alan Guttmacher Institute there were about 1.5 million abortions performed in 1992. During the days of illegal abortions many women died as a result of serious medical complications from these illegal abortions. In fact, the Institute of Medicine estimates this number to range between 1,000 and 10,000.[2] Often the abortions were performed by individuals who were inadequately skilled and working under unsanitary condi-

105

tions. Many other women suffered serious medical complications such as excessive bleeding, pelvic infections, and infertility.

Women today no longer have to resort to illegal abortions. Abortion has been legal in our country since 1973, when the Supreme Court decided in *Roe* v. *Wade* that a woman's constitutional right to privacy includes her right to decide if she wants to terminate her pregnancy. Since this decision, abortions are much safer and deaths and other serious complications from them are now extremely rare.

No matter what your age, you have the legal right to an abortion. However, if you are a minor there may be some restrictions to this right. The Supreme Court has ruled that states can require parental involvement with their daughter's decision if she is a minor. This means that, depending on your age, and depending on the laws in your state, your parents may need to be notified before you can have an abortion, or you may be required to get one or both of your parents' permission before getting an abortion. If you do not wish to involve your parents you must try to obtain a "judicial bypass." To do this, you must go to court and present your case before a judge. The judge will determine if you are mature enough to make your own decision to have an abortion.

If the judge decides you are mature enough, you can proceed with an abortion if you wish. However, the judge may decide that you are *not* mature enough to decide on your own. If this is the case, the judge will determine whether it's in your best interests to have an abortion. If you do not receive the judge's approval to have an abortion, you may appeal (go back to court to argue against the judge's decision). Your lawyer will help you with your appeal. According to the Planned Parenthood League of Massachusetts, since the laws requiring parental consent in Massachusetts went into effect in 1981, very few teens have been denied consent (judicial bypass) at their first hearing.[3]

Public Opinion

Abortion has become one of the most emotionally charged and controversial issues in our country. You may already be aware of this, or you may be confused about what people really think about abortion. Ever since the legalization of abortion, a battleground has been set up between two groups of individuals who have very different viewpoints. One group strongly opposes abortion, based on religious or moral reasons. This group is often referred to as "prolife." They feel that life begins at conception and believe abortion is murder. They believe that to end a life at any time is unacceptable and morally wrong. The other group strongly supports abortion, based on a woman's constitutional right to privacy which allows her to determine whether or not to terminate her pregnancy. This group is often referred to as "prochoice." They believe that a fetus really isn't a person, and feel that it is acceptable for a woman to choose to terminate her pregnancy under any circumstance. This group values a woman's own right to control when, and if, she wants a baby.

In recent years another, less vocal group of Americans has come forward with their views. Recent data indicate that this group supports a middle ground, that is, they support views from each side of the abortion debate. Researchers at Harvard University recently examined a hundred historical and current public opinion surveys about abortion. They found that this third group of individuals believe abortion is morally wrong, but they want abortion to remain legal.[4] They believe that abortion is a personal and private decision to be made by a woman with government only minimally involved. They feel abortion is acceptable under certain circumstances, such as when a woman's health is in jeopardy, or if the unborn child will suffer from serious birth defects, or in cases of rape. They do support some restrictions on a woman's private decision, such as requiring teens to notify a parent. There are circumstances in which they do not support legal abortion, such as when a family is poor, or a married woman does not want more children, or a single pregnant woman does not want to marry the father of her baby. They also do not believe that abortions should be paid for using public funds. These last several beliefs, especially regarding restricting access to abortion, are what separates this group from other prochoicers.

It's helpful to be aware of public opinions on abortion even if you don't agree with them. As you explore whether this option is right for you, it's likely that you will encounter someone who has strong views about abortion. This can happen to you with any of your options. You may talk to someone who doesn't believe a young woman should raise her baby or place her baby for adoption. It's good to be prepared for this. Everyone has a right to his or her own opinion. Whatever you decide to do is right for you. You do not have to accept someone else's opinion.

How Do Teens Feel about Abortion?

One study that looked at teen knowledge and attitudes about abortion found that many teens are confused and have misconceptions about abortion. Many teens mistakenly believe that abortion is dangerous and illegal and causes serious medical and emotional trauma to women. Even though many of the teens were concerned about a woman's health, most of the teens interviewed supported a woman's legal right to an abortion.

With all the controversy surrounding the abortion issue, it is no wonder that many teens are confused. *Terminating or ending your pregnancy is also referred to as abortion.* Abortion is a safe medical procedure. Even though there may be some restrictions on your ability to get an abortion because of parental notification or consent laws, you have the legal right to an abortion. *Abortion is not a form of birth control. Birth control measures block a pregnancy from happening; abortion terminates or ends a pregnancy after it has begun.* Many teens who are faced with an unintended pregnancy (a little more than one-third of all pregnant teens) choose to have an abortion.[5]

Choosing to have an abortion can be a difficult decision to make. There are moral, religious, and legal controversies surrounding the procedure. These controversies may or may not make it more difficult for you to make your decision. It's important for you to decide for yourself if abortion is the right choice for you. We believe that as long as abortion is legal you should be given as much information as possible so that you can feel comfortable making an informed decision for yourself. We hope that the information and resources provided here will help you with your decision-making process. *As with all your options, we strongly encourage you to involve your parents or another responsible adult with your decision process and plans.*

Having the legal right to an abortion provides you with reproductive freedom, which means that you can decide when, and whether or not, you want to have a baby. This freedom carries with it a lot of responsibility. It does not necessarily make your decision any easier. Deciding what you are going to do about your pregnancy is a serious choice. You must decide what the responsible thing for you to do is based on your own personal, moral, and religious beliefs. Right now at this point in your life your beliefs and values may not be clearly defined. You may be easily swayed by someone else's opinion. It's important for you to feel comfortable with whatever you decide to do. Your parents, family, boyfriend, and others close to you may all be affected in some way by whatever you decide to do, and will probably offer their advice. It's still your decision. It's important to think about what impact your decision will have on these people, as well as what you want for yourself at this point in your life, and the resources which are available to you right now.

Abortion has its advantages. If you view your pregnancy as a problem, an abortion is the easiest way to resolve your pregnancy. You will not have to continue your pregnancy and go through childbirth. You will not be faced with other difficult decisions to make, such as raising your baby, or placing your baby for adoption. You can go back to school and continue with your current life plans. Your friends and family don't need to know that you've had an abortion unless you choose to share this information with them.

Studies have revealed that teens who have an abortion tend to do better in many ways than teens who choose to raise their baby. One research study interviewed teens seeking pregnancy tests and compared those teens who had abortions with those who gave birth to their babies and those who had a negative pregnancy test.[6] Two years after the interview, the teens who had abortions had a more positive response. They were more likely to have stayed in school and graduated from high school and were less likely to have had another pregnancy during the two years than the teens who gave birth or whose pregnancy test was negative. The teens who chose abortion were better off financially than the other two groups. In addition the teens who chose abortion were no more likely to suffer stress or anxiety or have psychological problems two years later than the other two groups of teens.

Abortion has its disadvantages. If you choose to have an abortion you must make your decision in a short amount of time. Abortion is a serious decision to make, and you may feel rushed and uncomfortable making this decision in a limited amount of time. Abortion has the fewest medical complications when performed in the first trimester. A second trimester abortion can be performed, but there are limitations. There comes a point in time in your pregnancy in which an abortion is no longer possible. Second trimester abortions are more complicated procedures, but they are safe. They are more expensive, take longer to perform, and may require a hospital stay. What this means is that you need to make a serious decision quickly. The longer you wait the more expensive the procedure, the more emotionally attached you may become to your fetus, and the more you risk medical complications. Also, depending on what state you live in you may need to involve your parents. This may or may not be a problem for you. If you need your parents' consent and don't wish to involve them, you will have to deal with the legal system. Planned Parenthood or an abortion clinic can help you with this process. You will get confidential help usually at no cost to you; however, presenting your case to a judge may be an emotionally difficult experience for you and may cause a delay in getting your abortion.

There is a lot of public discussion today about the possible serious psychological problems women can suffer as a result of having an abortion. Prolife groups frequently cite findings from research studies to support their views that women do suffer psychological harm after having an abortion. Prochoice groups claim this isn't true. Who's right? In 1987, then Surgeon General of the United States C. Everett Koop was directed by President Ronald Reagan to study the health effects of abortion. Koop concluded that the research studies were flawed and did not provide conclusive evidence as to whether abortion does or does not cause psychological problems. He wrote that "at this time, the available scientific evidence about the psychological [consequences] of abortion simply cannot support either the preconceived beliefs of those [who are] prolife or those [who are] prochoice." In other words, right now, we can't be sure how a woman will react psychologically to having an abortion.[7]

Most people agree that everyone's emotional reaction to an abortion is different. Many young women who terminate an unintended pregnancy say they feel relieved afterwards. Others describe feelings of regret, sadness, or guilt. Some young women experience a greater sense of loss after their abortion if they had conflicting feelings and questioned whether or not they should have had the abortion in the first place. Feelings of loss are greater for young women who had an abortion when it was against their own values or beliefs and when they did not feel supported by their parents or partner. Young women who feel they have support for their decision and do not have conflicts over abortion are more satisfied with their decision afterward. Only you can evaluate what an abortion means to you and how much of an emotional loss you believe you will experience.

Reasons Why Teens Have Abortions

Deciding to have an abortion is a complex decision no matter how old you are. Sometimes a woman's pregnancy is very much desired, but for certain reasons she needs to have an abortion. For example, sometimes an abortion is performed because a woman has a disease and her pregnancy seriously jeopardizes her life. As discussed before, there are times when a woman chooses to have an abortion because her fetus is not healthy or may suffer from serious birth defects, and she wants to spare her baby a life of disability and suffering.

The majority of women who are faced with an unintended pregnancy make their decision to have an abortion based on a number of factors. Most young women feel they are too young and not ready to handle the responsibility of raising a baby. Many teens say that raising a baby would interfere with school or other personal plans they have. Many feel they can't afford to have a baby or they don't feel they have the support they need from their boyfriend or parents. One study found that young women had abortions for the following reasons:

- About three-fourths said they feared having a baby would totally change their lives in ways they weren't prepared for or didn't feel they could handle
- Two-thirds felt they could not afford to raise a baby
- One-half said they would be faced with raising a child alone and they did not want to do that
- About one-third felt they were not ready for the responsibility[8]

In chapter 8 you will read about Alison and Courtney. Alison was fourteen when she had her abortion. She felt she was too young and not emotionally ready to be a mother. She did not want to raise her baby alone, and was afraid that having a baby would interfere with school. This is what Alison had to say:

I considered myself much too young to be a mother and much too young to get married. Besides, John did not have the same feelings for me. . . . He wasn't willing to be a father at that point in his life. It would not have been impossible for me to care for my baby while I was in school . . . [but] I knew I just wasn't ready to be a mother. Emotionally I didn't have it in me to be a mother. . . . Having a baby at age fourteen was not the way I always dreamed my life would turn out. I planned to go to college first, get married, then have kids.

Courtney was in college when she had her first abortion. She describes several factors which influenced her decision: she was fearful of what her friends and parents would think of her pregnancy; she would have also been faced with raising her child on her own, which she didn't feel she was emotionally ready to do. Courtney said:

I was afraid of my parents' reaction and I didn't want to have to tell them of my pregnancy. . . . I knew my parents expected me to finish college,

although I also knew that being Catholic, they would expect me to marry.
. . . I wanted to have a career as well as finish college. I was not ready emotionally or financially to raise a child or to get married. Even though I was
in love with Steve, despite his limitations, it did not feel like I was ready
for marriage. . . . I felt my friends would abandon me because I was careless and stupid enough to allow myself to become pregnant. . . . I would
have been ashamed to be a single, pregnant girl. . . . I couldn't comprehend
living out that scenario.

Another young woman describes the frustration of what it's like to want
to raise your baby, but to feel that you can't afford to raise your baby. This
is how Kara described her situation:

I was a teen parent with one child already. I enjoyed being a mom. But, I
was trying my hardest to break away from the cycle of poverty. I couldn't
afford to have another baby. It wasn't fair to my first child or to my unborn
baby. Having the abortion meant survival for myself and my family. I don't
regret my decision. It was the right thing for me to do in my situation. I feel
it's wrong to have a child when you can't properly take care of it.

Jenny describes what her life was like when she became pregnant and
how that had an impact on her decision to have an abortion. Jenny said:

I was seventeen when I got pregnant. I didn't intend to. I had always told
myself that if I got pregnant, I would do the responsible thing and raise my
baby. But when I found myself in that situation I decided to have an abortion instead. At first I was very uncertain about my decision, but then I
came to realize that it was the best thing for me to do. At the time I was in
therapy. My mother and I were always fighting. I didn't know how to speak
up for myself. My boyfriend and I had just broken up. I realized there were
too many things in my life which I had to deal with first before having a
baby. Because I had so many unresolved issues with my mother, I decided
it would be more emotionally traumatic for me to become a mother now
than it would to have an abortion.

The decision to have an abortion was difficult for Shannon to make. She
was raised Catholic and didn't feel she could continue her pregnancy and
raise her baby or place her baby for adoption. This is what Shannon said:

Initially I struggled with my decision. I'm Catholic, I didn't believe in abortion but at sixteen I didn't feel capable of being a mother. I didn't feel I could

continue my pregnancy and then place my baby for adoption. There was too much going on in my home. My dad lost his job. He was drinking too much and could get verbally abusive if it was a bad day. My mom was working two jobs to try to support us all and seemed to be on the verge of a nervous breakdown from all the stress. It would have been too much of an emotional ordeal for me to continue my pregnancy under those circumstances. In the end, although it was against my religious beliefs, I felt it was better for me to have an abortion. I made the decision with my boyfriend. I went to court so that I did not have to tell my parents or get their permission. I was afraid of what my dad would do if he found out about my pregnancy.

Decision-Making Process

Choosing to have an abortion is a deeply personal decision. The decision process is complex. There are many different factors which may influence your decision. Some women find it an emotionally difficult decision to make, and some do not. Some teens know for sure that they want an abortion. They see abortion as a positive choice, as the best way for them to resolve an unintended pregnancy. Like Jenny, they feel it would be more emotionally traumatic for them to continue their pregnancy. Other young women struggle with their decision because of their own religious beliefs, or the religious beliefs of someone close to them. Shannon initially struggled with her decision because of religious beliefs, but then was able to resolve this issue and felt comfortable with her decision to have an abortion.

The emotions each woman experiences about her pregnancy and her reasons for wanting to terminate her pregnancy are her own unique reasons. Women who have carefully made their decision and have support from their family and boyfriend report a feeling of relief after the abortion. They may feel sad about their abortion, but they tend not to regret what they did, or experience long-term emotional trauma. It's important for you to take the time to carefully consider this option, along with all your other options. Each woman's life experience is different. You are the only person who knows what your needs are, what your current situation is like, and which option is best for you. You will have to live with your decision. The following questions may help you to decide if abortion is the best option for you:

Is this your decision, or did someone else make the decision for you?

In chapter 3 you read about Yolanda, who told her mom that she was pregnant and was shocked to find out that her mom insisted she have an abortion or live elsewhere. Yolanda didn't know what to do. She did not want to have an abortion, so she turned to an aunt for help. She was able to live at her aunt's home and raise her baby there. In chapter 9, you will read about Carolyn, whose boyfriend pressured her to have an abortion. Carolyn did not want to have an abortion because it was against her religious beliefs. She made the decision which she felt was right for her. She continued her pregnancy and placed her baby for adoption. Her relationship didn't last with her boyfriend. Today she's happy. She's in college, and she's dating someone else. Most of all she has peace of mind. Her baby is being raised in a loving family, and she did what was best for herself and her child.

Some women feel pressure to have an abortion just like Yolanda and Carolyn did. Abortion to some people is an easy solution to an unintended pregnancy. It has to be your decision to have an abortion. No one should force you to have an abortion against your will.

Have you thoroughly thought through all your options?

It's important to carefully consider all your options before you make a final decision. Abortion is a permanent response; once you have an abortion you cannot undo your actions. Remember, there are other options besides abortion. You can continue your pregnancy and either raise your baby or place your baby for adoption. Today both of these options are socially acceptable. There are people to whom you can talk who can help you decide which option is best for you. Carefully considering all your options now will help prevent you from having self-doubts and regrets later on in your life. This will be discussed with you in your preabortion counseling.

Courtney made her decision alone, at a time when she felt panic and fear. She knew she wasn't capable of raising her baby at that time in her life; however, she never considered adoption. Having an abortion caused her to feel a real loss which she struggled with at the time and which she still has not fully resolved. She wishes she had sought help with her decision making because she feels that if she had, she would have chosen to do something different. She believes now that adoption would have been a better choice for her.

What does abortion mean to you?

By now you are aware of what abortion means to the general public as well as to some other teens. Unfortunately, with the decision you are about to make other people's opinions don't count. No one else can advise whether abortion is right for you. It may help you to know that others share some of the same feelings you have, and have gone through similar circumstances. However, abortion is *your* decision to make; no one else can make it for you. It's important to take the time to explore what abortion means to you. If at this time you feel abortion is best for you but you have some lingering doubts because of religious or other reasons, try to resolve them before you have an abortion. It's easier to resolve these feelings now while you still have other options to pursue. Find someone you trust with whom you can sort out your feelings. If you do something which is against your values, beliefs, or instincts you may be angry with yourself later on and may experience a greater emotional loss.

If you are considering abortion, but are concerned because abortion conflicts with your religious values, it may help you to know that there are members within various religions who support a woman's right to decide whether she wants to terminate her pregnancy. A list of these organizations is included at the end of the book. You may also want to talk about this some more with someone from your church, keeping in mind that teachings about abortion vary.

Have you thought about what the emotional loss will be for you?
Regardless of which option you choose, you will experience an emotional loss. A pregnancy is a major life event, especially at this time in your life. Experiencing loss is normal and a healthy way of processing what has happened to you. Choosing abortion does not necessarily mean that you will not experience a loss. Some women view an abortion as their best choice and feel it is less traumatic for them than raising a baby. That's okay. No one can tell you that you have to feel remorse, regret, or guilt about your decision. Other women, such as Courtney, had an abortion and didn't realize that they would experience a loss later on in their life. Courtney has struggled with her loss for many years, and still has not resolved it. Think very carefully about all your decisions and the loss you might experience with each option before you decide to have an abortion.

THINGS TO CONSIDER

Below are some important points of which you should be aware as you are deciding if abortion is right for you. If you choose abortion you need to make a decision fairly quickly. These points should help you stay on track while you're making your decision.

- Don't make a hasty decision, but try to make your decision as soon as possible. Abortions are safer and less expensive when done during the first trimester of a pregnancy. Even if you make your decision when you are six weeks pregnant, it may take you additional time to come up with the money, book an appointment, or get consent if needed in your state.
- It's your decision to make, even though the people you are close to will be affected by your decision and may try to influence what you do. No one should force you to have an abortion against your will.
- If you're considering abortion and don't want to involve your parents, find out right away what your state laws are regarding notification and parental consent. If notification or parental consent is required and you do not intend to get permission from your parents, you will have to go to court. This may take extra time. Try to plan for this early so you don't have to delay your abortion. A delay in your abortion may cause you to have a second trimester abortion, which is more complicated, has more risks, and is more expensive.
- At all times protect your health. If you decide to have an abortion, make sure you have a legal and safe abortion.
- If you want an abortion and can't afford one, there may be financial resources available for you. You can call different abortion clinics to find out what is available to you.

Planned Parenthood is one resource available to you. Call your local Planned Parenthood office for help with pregnancy testing, pregnancy counseling, information on your state's parental notification or consent laws, assistance with the consent process if it is needed, referral for abortion, prenatal care, adoption services, or referral for financial assistance whether you are terminating your pregnancy or continuing it. To find the nearest Planned Parenthood, call 1–800–230–PLAN, or look under your local Yellow Pages under "Birth Control Information Centers" or "Clinics."

You can also get referral information from the National Abortion Federation Hotline. The telephone number is (800) 772–9100.

WHEN CAN AN ABORTION BE PERFORMED?

The Supreme Court has ruled that abortions are legal for all women in this country. There are times, however, when states can regulate (in other words, limit) when one can have an abortion. States cannot prohibit a woman's right to have an abortion during the first trimester of pregnancy. States can restrict a woman's right to have an abortion after the first trimester in order to protect the health of the pregnant woman, or to protect fetal life after viability. Viability refers to a point in time between conception and birth in which the fetus can survive outside of the mother's body. This happens near the end of the second trimester. This means you can have an abortion up until about the middle of the second trimester. However, it's best not to put off having an abortion that long. Abortions, although safe in the second trimester, are safer and less expensive if done in the first trimester. Second trimester abortions are more costly, take longer, and have an increased risk of complications. According to the Alan Guttmacher Institute, the majority of all abortions in this country are performed during the first trimester. However, teens are more likely than older women to have second trimester abortions. This is probably related to the fact that many teens do not realize they are pregnant, delay making a decision, or have to go to court and get a judge's permission prior to having their abortion if parental permission is not going to be obtained.

HOW IS AN ABORTION PERFORMED?

FIRST TRIMESTER ABORTION

The majority of first trimester abortions are performed using the *vacuum aspiration* method. This is a simple and safe technique which can be performed in a doctor's office or clinic using local anesthesia (a medication which affects only the cervix). You may be able to request varying types of anesthesia so that you can be awake, sedated (drowsy), or asleep. Local anesthesia carries the least risk.

A local anesthetic similar to novocaine is injected and numbs the cervix. After injecting the anesthetic, the doctor first dilates or widens the cervix, and then inserts a small flexible tube through the opening and into the uterus. This small tube is attached to a suction machine which then draws out the contents of the uterus. During the procedure you may not feel anything at all, or you may experience anything from mild menstrual-like cramps to a fair amount of cramping. The doctor will then check the tissue in order to be certain that the contents of the uterus have been completely removed. The entire procedure lasts five to seven minutes. There is an additional thirty-five to forty-five minutes of recovery time, in which you will be monitored by clinic personnel for any signs of complications. This procedure can be performed through thirteen weeks of pregnancy.[9] Your doctor will take into consideration the size of your uterus and your last menstrual period (LMP) to determine how far into the pregnancy you are. Often the determination is made by ultrasound, a picture of the contents of the uterus; this adds to the cost of the procedure but is necessary when the length of the pregnancy is unclear.

The procedure requires only local anesthesia. Many women do well with only a local anesthetic. However, some women want to be asleep during the procedure. If you want to be asleep, you can request general anesthesia. You won't see what's happening or feel pain. If you receive general anesthesia the abortion will be more expensive and the recovery time will be longer. General anesthesia is not available at all abortion clinics. If you feel strongly that you need to be asleep during the procedure you may have to shop around to find an abortion clinic which offers general anesthesia. In some places you can have intravenous medication (drugs injected into your vein) in combination with a local anesthetic. You won't be completely asleep, but this will help you feel more relaxed and sedated during the procedure. If you have trouble with pain or are very anxious, this may be a good option for you. There is also an extra fee for this option, and it may take longer to recover.

The medical risks associated with anesthesia increase with the amount of anesthesia used. This doesn't mean you need to suffer; however, more is not necessarily better. *Any concerns you have regarding any part of the procedure should be directed to the clinic physician.*

SECOND TRIMESTER ABORTION

There are varying methods used for second trimester abortions. Second trimester abortions are more complicated because the pregnancy is more advanced and the fetus is much larger. They involve more health risks, can be emotionally more difficult for you, and are more expensive.

Dilation and Evacuation (also called D&E) is a method used for abortions up to twenty-one weeks. This is a two-day process. The cervix needs to be dilated more because larger instruments are needed. The first day, laminaria sticks are inserted into the cervical opening. These are sterile seaweed sticks that gradually dilate or expand the cervix overnight, so that on the second day the cervix will be wide enough for the procedure. The doctor injects the cervix with a local anesthetic, and then dilators are used to gradually widen the cervix even more. The doctor then uses special instruments along with vacuum suction to remove the contents of the uterus. The procedure takes longer than a first trimester abortion, about fifteen to twenty-five minutes to complete.

An *induced abortion* is another type of second trimester abortion. It is more complicated, needs to be done in a hospital, and a twelve- to twenty-four-hour hospital stay may be required. This will be expensive. The doctor injects a solution through the abdomen and into the amniotic sac which surrounds the fetus. You will experience labor and delivery. Pain relief is provided throughout this process and a dilation and curettage (D&C) often follows delivery to insure that the uterus is completely empty.*

The type of anesthesia used for second trimester abortion depends on the facility you go to; each has its own policies. *Any concerns you have about anesthesia or the procedure should be directed to the clinic physician.*

HOW SAFE IS AN ABORTION?

Abortion is one of the most commonly performed surgical procedures in this country. As with any surgical procedure, there are potential medical risks, but the medical risks of legal abortion appear to be very small. The risk of a woman dying from a legal abortion today is very low. According to the Guttmacher Institute, less than 1 percent of women having abortions experience a major complication as a result of the procedure.[11] The chances of developing a complication increase the later in the pregnancy the abortion is performed. Teenagers do not appear to be at a higher risk of developing serious complications from abortions than are older women. Complications related to an abortion procedure include pelvic infection, hemorrhage (abnormal bleeding), uterine perforation (a tear in the uterus), and injury to the cervix. You should notify your doctor if you start to bleed heavily, have a fever or chills, become very weak, have abdominal pain or cramping, or a foul-smelling vaginal discharge after an abortion. These are all symptoms which may indicate that you are experiencing a medical complication and require medical attention.

Many young women are concerned that their ability to have a baby in the future will be affected. This is a normal concern to have. You should discuss this concern as well as the potential medical risks with your abortion provider prior to your abortion. Recent research suggests that a vacuum

---

*Recall that a D&C is sometimes performed after a miscarriage to ensure that the contents of the uterus are completely removed. A D&C is very similar to the D&E just described, but the D&C does not use any vacuum suction to empty the uterus. Instead, the physician performs this task manually, using instruments known as curettes to carefully scrape clean the inside walls of the uterus.

aspiration abortion performed in the first trimester has little effect on a woman's future fertility, but there are no guarantees.

Where Can I Go?

The majority of first trimester abortions are performed in clinics that function independently and are not part of hospitals. Abortions can also be performed in doctors' offices, outpatient departments, and hospitals. Abortions performed in hospitals are much more expensive and it is not usually necessary to have a first trimester abortion in a hospital setting. Your doctor may advise you to have an abortion in a hospital if you have a serious medical condition which may put you more at risk of complications, or if you are having a second trimester abortion. Some abortion clinics are equipped to safely perform a second trimester abortion, but most are not. If there is none in your area, you may have to travel to find one.

To locate a reliable abortion provider in your area you can call your local Planned Parenthood office. You can also call the National Abortion Federation Hotline, (800) 772–9100, or look in the Yellow Pages under "Abortion Providers." Your health care provider, local family planning clinic, or neighborhood health center may also be able to refer you to a reliable abortion provider. *Shop around for a reliable abortion provider. Do not rely on your girlfriends' advice.*

You should also be aware of "crisis pregnancy centers." These centers, often operated by prolife groups, provide pregnancy testing, counseling, and assistance to women who choose to continue their pregnancies.

What Can I Expect?

No matter where you go for an abortion, you are entitled to be treated with respect and dignity. As one nurse from an abortion clinic said:

> It's important for you to feel comfortable wherever you choose to go. Many clinics are staffed with people who like to help people. They are very sensitive to the needs of the women they serve. They take pride in their work. They are there to help you, and you can trust that they will maintain your privacy and confidentiality.

Unfortunately all providers are not the same, and you may come across someone who is insensitive or not supportive. This can make your experience uncomfortable for you.

You should also prepare yourself for potential protesters who may be in front of the clinic demonstrating against abortions when you arrive. The pro-life movement is very vocal in some communities. You should understand there may be prolife groups there. You may want to call the clinic first to find out if there are times when these groups are less likely to be present. Usually these protesters are not out to hurt anyone. They feel strongly about their views, and they want the opportunity to express them. If you are confronted by protesters, it's best to ignore them and continue walking. Don't talk back to them. This will only frustrate you more. You can't change their minds. Their beliefs and opinions are their own. They do not have to be yours.

QUESTIONS TO ASK

Abortion providers are not all alike. Providers vary by the types of services they offer and their cost. For instance, some providers perform first trimester abortions only, and some are equipped to perform both first and second trimester abortions. The following is a list of questions to ask each provider as you're deciding which provider to go to:

- What are the parental consent laws or other laws in my state of which I need to be aware? If I need my parents' permission and I do not want to tell them, will you help me with the court process? Can you provide me a lawyer? Do I have to pay for the lawyer? Will this service be confidential?
- What is the cost of the procedure? Is everything included, or will there be other charges? If I can't afford the abortion, can you help me find a way to pay for it?
- What type of abortion will be performed? What types of anesthesia or other medications are available? What are the medical or other risks I should be aware of?
- Will I have an opportunity to discuss my feelings first with a counselor or nurse? Will someone be with me during the procedure?
- Can I bring someone with me?
- How long should I expect to be there? How will I feel when I leave?
- Will you provide any follow-up care that I may need? If so, what is the cost?
- Are there demonstrators there blocking the entrance? If so, do you do anything to intervene?

This list is just a beginning. Feel free to ask any question you have so that you feel comfortable with the abortion provider you choose.

WHAT ARE MY LEGAL RIGHTS?

If you are a minor, your parents are legally responsible for you. Depending on your age and your relationship with your parents, this may bother you. You may be feeling independent and wanting to take more responsibility for matters that are important to you, such as getting an abortion. Usually your parents must be notified or give their permission before you can receive most medical treatment, but parental notification or consent laws vary from state to state. Usually state laws allow teens to consent to their own health care in certain situations, such as treatment of sexually transmitted diseases, prenatal care, family planning, or care related to substance abuse. Any provider you go to should be aware of these laws and be able to explain to you what your state laws mean for you regarding each of these circumstances. If you feel you are not getting adequate advice you can call your local Planned Parenthood. You may be able to get additional information from your local legal aid office or another legal advocacy group.

The issue of parental notification or consent before a minor can have an abortion is a very sensitive public policy issue. Public opinion polls show that even though the majority of voters favor legalized abortion, they strongly support parental notification or consent laws before minors' abortions. Many believe parental notification or consent laws are in the teens' best interest. All teens differ in their emotional needs and ability to make a decision. Many feel that parents' involvement will only benefit teens. Parents know their daughter's emotional needs and would be better able to provide her with emotional support and guidance, as well as protect her from any harm. There are others who feel strongly that teens are capable of making their own decision, and fear that parental notification and consent laws act as barriers which delay or prevent a teen from getting an abortion.

Many states currently have mandatory parental notification or consent laws, and it's likely that these laws will remain in effect for some time. This means that depending on the laws in your state, and depending on your age, one or both of your parents may need to be notified and/or give consent before you have an abortion. If the state in which you live has either a parental notification or consent law, your state must provide you with an opportunity to appear before a judge and demonstrate that you are mature enough to make your own decision without your parent's notification or consent. This is also known as a judicial bypass process. Most abortion providers assist minors through this process by helping them find a lawyer at no cost who will be with them when they appear before the judge.

SHOULD I TELL MY PARENTS?

Only you know for sure what the answer is to this question. Parental notification and consent laws were designed to protect a young woman's best interests. Deciding to have an abortion is a big decision. All young women differ in their ability to make a decision. This may be the biggest decision you have ever made and you may be distressed by it, or you may feel quite comfortable in your ability to make an important decision such as this one. It turns out that, even when parental notification or consent laws do not require it, many young women do tell one of their parents, usually their mother, before they have an abortion.

One recent study which was conducted in states without mandatory parental notification and consent laws found the following:

- 61 percent of the pregnant teens reported that one or both of their parents knew of their abortion and the majority of the parents supported their daughter's decision to have an abortion.
- 78 percent of the pregnant teens involved their boyfriend in making the decision or getting the abortion.
- The pregnant teens who did not inform their parents didn't do so because they worried that it would hurt their relationship or they feared their parents' disappointment, anger, or adding to their stress.[12]

Alison was fearful of telling her dad. She was worried about adding to his stress. He had a lot going on at work and her parents had just gone through a difficult divorce. She found out that her dad was glad she came to him and he was supportive of her decision. She was able to get the help she needed to make her decision and arrange for the abortion.

Shannon, whose situation was different from Alison's, decided to go to court rather than risk telling her parents about her pregnancy and trying to get their permission. Shannon was also fearful of increasing the stress in her home. She feared her father would be angry, and she worried about how he would react. If you've never been to a doctor alone before, or if you've never had a surgical procedure done alone before, this may be scary and intimidating for you. *We strongly encourage you to involve your parent or, if you do not feel you can, to involve another older, responsible adult in your decision-making process.* The more emotional support and guidance you have the more comfortable you will feel with your decision.

Loss Associated with Abortion

You will experience a loss no matter which option you choose. The extent of the loss you feel will depend on your personal circumstances. Each woman's emotional response to an abortion is different. Many young women describe feeling relieved after their abortion. However, some young women describe feelings of sadness, guilt, regret, and anger. Usually these feelings are short-term and subside with time as a young woman processes her loss and resumes her life.

You may recall the study presented in the beginning of this chapter which compared teens who had abortions to teens who gave birth and to teens who had a negative pregnancy test. This particular study showed that two years later, the teens who had the abortions were doing much better than the other two groups. They were more likely to be on track with their education and were financially better off. Most important, they were no more likely to have psychological problems than the other two groups of teens.[13]

Women who have a harder time making their decision to terminate their pregnancy are more likely to experience a greater sense of loss after their abortion. One study found that women who had difficulty several days before deciding to have an abortion reported negative feelings two to three months after the abortion.[14] Women who have second trimester abortions also report more emotional distress after abortion than do those women who have first trimester abortions.

Women who feel they have more support for their decision from their parents and boyfriend and who do not have negative attitudes about abortion are more satisfied with their decision. It seems that young women who make a decision alone, who hold negative views about abortion, and who do not have support for their decision from their parents and/or boyfriend are less satisfied with their decision and experience more emotional distress.

Being honest with yourself, exploring all your options and making a careful decision after speaking with an older, responsible adult will increase the likelihood that you will make a decision that works for you. You have to live with your decision now and in years to come. If you have an abortion now and it's contrary to your values, you may regret your decision later on and experience a greater degree of loss.

SUGGESTIONS FOR COPING WITH LOSS

- Don't be too hard on yourself. Recognize that you made the decision you believe is best for yourself at this time in your life.
- Have fun. Get more involved in life. Take up a new hobby or a new sport. Any form of regular exercise can help to decrease any stress that you may be feeling.
- Spend more time with your friends. Develop new relationships.
- Use what happened as a valuable learning experience. Take some time to learn more about yourself, what your limitations are, what kinds of relationships you want with boyfriends, and what you want out of life.
- Keep a journal. Writing can be a great outlet for your feelings.
- Reproductive freedom means reproductive responsibility. If you plan on being sexually active, speak to your health care provider and select and use a contraceptive method that will work for you. Remember, *hope is not a contraceptive method.*
- Give yourself permission to grieve. Don't deny your feelings. Let people know how you feel. If your feelings of stress or sadness continue, get some help. There may be something going on in your life in addition to your abortion which is troubling you and which you need to resolve.

Notes

1. Institute of Medicine, *The Best Intentions. Unintended Pregnancy and the Well-Being of Children and Families* (Washington, D.C.: National Academy Press, 1995), p. 51.

2. Ibid.

3. Planned Parenthood League of Massachusetts, "Consent for Abortion: What Women under 18 Need to Know" (pamphlet) (Cambridge: Planned Parenthood League of Massachusetts, n.d.).

4. R. J. Blendon, J. M. Benson, and K. Donelan, "The Public and the Controversy over Abortion," *Journal of the American Medical Association* 270, no. 23 (1993): 2871–75.

5. The Alan Guttmacher Institute, "Abortion in the United States," *Facts in Brief* (pamphlet) (New York: Alan Guttmacher Institute, 1995).

6. L. S. Zabin, M. B. Hirsch, and M. R. Emerson, "When Urban Adolescents Choose Abortion: Effects on Education, Psychological Status and Subsequent Pregnancy," *Family Planning Perspectives* 21, no. 6 (1989): 248–55.

7. C. E. Koop, "A Measured Response: Koop on Abortion," *Family Planning Perspectives* 21, no. 1 (1989): 31–32.

8. A. Torres and J. D. Forrest, "Why Do Women Have Abortions?" *Family Planning Perspectives* 20, no. 4 (1988): 169–76.

9. The American College of Obstetricians and Gynecologists, *PRECIS V: An Update in Obstetrics and Gynecology* (Washington, D.C.: ACOG, 1994), p. 291.

10. Ibid., p. 293.

11. Guttmacher Institute, "Abortion in the United States."

12. S. K. Henshaw and K. Kost, "Parental Involvement in Minors' Abortion Decisions," *Family Planning Perspectives* 24, no. 5 (1992): 196–207, 213.

13. Zabin, Hirsch, and Emerson, "When Urban Adolescents Choose Abortion."

14. N. E. Adler, "Emotional Responses of Women Following Therapeutic Abortion," *American Journal of Orthopsychiatry* 45, no. 3 (1975): 446–54.

6

Considering Adoption?

To thine own self be true.

William Shakespeare

Adoption has always been an option for women who feel they are not ready to parent. Since biblical times women have placed their children in the loving care of others. Moses, one of the most famous biblical leaders, was adopted. Other people you might know who were adopted include John J. Audubon (naturalist), Shari Belafonte-Harper (actress), Senator Robert Byrd, Peter and Kitty Carruthers and Scott Hamilton (ice-skaters), Nat King Cole (singer), Faith Daniels (television news personality), Ted Danson (actor), Eric Dickerson (professional football player), President Gerald Ford, Steven Paul Jobs (founder of Apple Computers), Charlotte Anne Lopez (Miss Teen USA), Marilyn Monroe (actress), Jim Palmer (professional baseball player), and Nancy Reagan (former First Lady). The list goes on and on.[1]

Adoption is another way to form a family. It is the legal placement of a child with an individual or couple who will raise the child as their own. The biological parents are comforted knowing that someone will provide a secure, loving home for their child. Adopted children are lovingly cared for by their adoptive parents. They become a legal member of the adoptive family in every possible way, including the right to a full inheritance. The adoptive parents are able to fulfill their dream of raising a child. The love

127

they have for their adopted child is the same love a parent has for any child in their family.

Throughout history, children who were separated from their biological parents for any number of reasons have become legally adopted by another family. In Moses' case, his biological mother, a Hebrew woman, feared for his survival. At that time in history the king of Egypt had ordered that all Hebrew boys be killed. When Moses was three months old and his mother could no longer hide him she placed him in a basket and left him in the reeds by the river bank, hoping to protect him from the king. The king's daughter found him, and even though he was a Hebrew child, she adopted him as her son. Placing a baby for adoption can be a difficult decision to make. A young woman considers what's best for her child's welfare and makes a loving and caring decision.

Over the years, millions of people have been adopted, and it is likely that millions more will be adopted, although the actual number of adoptees in this country is not known because national statistics on adoption are not maintained. One survey by the National Council for Adoption found that in 1986 there were 51,157 unrelated adoptions of American children. These were legal adoptions by people who were not biologically related to the adopted child; in other words, this number does not include relative or step-parent adoptions. About one-half of the 51,157 were adoptions of healthy infants and children under two years of age who were of all races and ethnic backgrounds. One way to estimate the number of adoptees in this country who are currently seventy-five years old or younger is to multiply the number of adoptees in 1986 by seventy-five, which equals 3,836,775.* That's a lot of people who are adopted. It's very likely that you know someone who is adopted. An even more important figure is the number of potential adoptive parents. The National Council for Adoption estimates that there are between one and two million infertile and fertile couples, as well as individuals, who are interested in adopting a child. If you choose to place your baby for adoption you can be comforted knowing that there are many potential adoptive parents.

Adoption is not as common today as it was years ago. Many teens are choosing to parent their child or to terminate their pregnancy. Young women today have more options than women did in the 1950s and 1960s when

---

*This is just a rough estimate because the adoption rates change somewhat from year to year (for example, more adoptions occurred in the 1950s and 1960s than in recent years), but it gives you a general idea.

adoption was more common. Back then, abortion was illegal and single parenthood was not as socially acceptable as it is today. When a young, single woman became pregnant, she usually married the father of her baby. However, marriage was not always a possibility. Very few single women raised their babies. They worried that they would be punished by society for their actions. More often, a young pregnant woman had an illegal abortion or placed her baby for adoption. Because it was socially unacceptable to be a single parent and because you had to risk your health to have an illegal abortion, many young women felt forced to place their child for adoption.

Times have changed. Abortion is now legal and safe. It's more socially acceptable for a young woman to raise her child on her own. A young, unmarried woman is no longer expected to place her child for adoption. Today, adoption is a deliberate choice: A young woman chooses adoption because she feels it's best for her baby and herself.

Why Teens Choose Adoption

There are many reasons why a young woman chooses adoption. Because of religious or personal beliefs a young woman may not want to have an abortion, or she may have waited too long to have an abortion. Young women who choose adoption do so because they are concerned about the potential negative consequences of early parenting for both their children and themselves. They are concerned about their ability to be a good parent. Most young women who choose this option are single. They don't feel they have the emotional or financial resources to parent their child. A young woman may want to delay parenting until she's married, and marriage may not be a possibility for her at this time. The young woman may feel she's too young to get married. She may not be sure that her boyfriend is the person with whom she wants to spend the rest of her life. Her boyfriend may not be interested in marriage or in helping her raise her child.

Because they have limited financial resources, young women know they will need to rely on their families for help. They worry about the financial strain that this will place on their families. Many young women want to complete their education and establish their careers before they become mothers. In addition, young women who choose adoption have a more positive view about adoption than the young women who choose to have abortions or parent their children. Oftentimes they may have been adopted themselves or have a family member or friend who was adopted.

Adoption for most young women is not a quick decision. Young women who choose adoption take time to consult with their parents, boyfriend, friends, and other adults. In the end they make their decision because they feel it's in the best interest of their baby and themselves. Amy placed her baby for adoption. She explains why she chose this option:

> I don't believe in abortion. I also don't feel I'm ready to be a mother yet. I haven't even finished high school. I want a career and to be married before I have a family. I'm too young to know if the father of my baby is the man I want to be with for the rest of my life. He's the first guy I've ever dated. Right now he's not willing to help raise our child. My child deserves better. I want my child to have a father and mother who are ready to be parents.

Marianna also chose to place her baby for adoption. She felt it was best for her baby, herself, and her family. She didn't have her boyfriend's support. Marianna explains:

> For religious reasons, I don't believe in abortion. I love children, but I couldn't see how I could realistically care for my baby. My boyfriend Ricky and I had broken up. I'd have to rely on my parents to support us, and they don't have a lot of money. They each have jobs. We live in a small two-bedroom house. My older sister and I share the same room. On top of that, my mother had a baby last year. My baby sister stays with my parents now in their bedroom. When she gets bigger she's going to need her space. There's not enough room. My parents work hard simply to get by. I couldn't put them through any more stress. I love them too much. It just wouldn't be fair to them. I chose to place my baby for adoption. This is something I feel good about.

Joan is another young women who placed her baby for adoption. She didn't feel she was emotionally ready to be a parent. She wasn't sure if she ever wanted to be a mother. Here's what Joan said:

> I was sexually abused by my uncle when I was a child. It's something that I haven't dealt with and it still haunts me to this day. I placed my baby for adoption because I knew I wasn't emotionally ready to be a parent. The way I look at it right now, I'm not so sure I'll ever want to be a mother. I have too many bad memories of my childhood.

Carolyn, who tells her story in chapter 9, placed her baby for adoption because she wanted to establish a career before she had a family. She held positive views about adoption. This is what Carolyn said:

I thought about all my options over and over. I knew it would be difficult to raise a child even with my parents' help. I wanted to go to college and have a career. I had always dreamed of living in a foreign country before settling down and having children. I began to think more and more about adoption. My cousin was adopted. We are the same age. She has a good relationship with her parents, my aunt and uncle. She told me she wonders why her birth mother placed her for adoption, but she doesn't spend a lot of time thinking about it. She just figures her mother couldn't raise her by herself and wanted her to have two parents.

Young women who receive comprehensive pregnancy counseling are more likely to choose adoption than young women who do not receive this service. One recent research study which evaluated the decision-making process of pregnant teens who chose adoption revealed the following:

- Pregnant teens who received pregnancy counseling which included information on adoption were seven times more likely to choose adoption than pregnant teens who received counseling which did not include adoption.
- Pregnant teens who involved their parents with their decision-making process were six times more likely to choose adoption than those who did not involve their parents.
- Pregnant teens who were asked to think about how their lives would change if they parented versus if they chose adoption were six times more likely to choose adoption than pregnant teens who did not make these comparisons.[2]

Why Teens Don't Choose Adoption

Today fewer teens are considering adoption. One possible explanation is that young women now have more options from which to choose. Instead of choosing adoption as young women would have done years ago, modern teens are choosing to parent their child or terminate their pregnancy. In order to better understand these changes, one researcher recently studied the attitudes toward adoption among pregnant teens and others whom the teens identified as influential in their decision-making process. She concluded that pregnant teens are usually aware that adoption is an option, but they do not choose it for the following reasons: fear of societal sanctions, inaccurate knowledge about adoption, anticipated difficulty coping with the emotional pain, and lack of support from helping professionals.[3]

Because it is more socially acceptable today to be a single parent, many teens mistakenly worry that it is socially unacceptable to place their baby for adoption. Many teens overwhelmingly believe that the responsible thing to do is to parent their child. Unfortunately, some pregnant teens do not find support for adoption within their community. Some feel pressure to raise their child from their parents, boyfriends, and friends. Sally said, "I got pregnant. I'm being responsible. I'm caring for my baby. My family always told me to be responsible for my mistakes. It wouldn't be right for me to expect someone else to do it."

Another pregnant teen was encouraged by her mother, sisters, and boyfriend to raise her baby. She feels she no longer has their support, which upsets her. Here's what Anna said:

> I kept my baby because everyone told me to. My boyfriend told me there was no way he was going to let me give my baby away. My baby is almost a year old. We need a lot of help. All of a sudden no one's there for me anymore. I'm on my own. It's been really tough.

Many pregnant teens lack accurate knowledge about adoption. In one study, only three out of twenty-one teens interviewed had any accurate information about adoption.[4] Most of the teens did not receive adoption information or counseling during their pregnancy. Another study found that persons providing counseling were even less informed about adoption and/or were reluctant to talk about adoption based on an assumption that pregnant teens would have no interest in it as an option.[5] Some health care providers are hesitant to discuss adoption because they are fearful that they may alienate you from receiving health care. It's normal to be hesitant about choosing an option if you're not given information on it. You may have to speak up or pursue adoption counseling from other sources if you don't feel you're getting the advice you need. Other research has shown that pregnant teens benefit from pregnancy counseling which includes information on adoption. Teens who received adoption counseling were much more likely to choose adoption.

Fear of long term emotional pain was the most powerful reason why pregnant teens did not choose adoption in one research study. Many of the teens interviewed worried that they would experience guilt, ongoing grief, and concern that their child would always hate them for the decision they made. Janet expresses similar feelings about adoption:

> I carried my baby for nine months. I had morning sickness, put on a lot of weight, and felt her kick and move. After going through all that, there's no

way I could let anyone else raise my child. That would be too painful for me. I couldn't handle that.

As with any decision you choose, you will experience a loss. The loss you will experience from adoption is a loss which you can handle with support and counseling and it will lessen in time. One recent research study which compared pregnant teens who chose adoption with single teens who parented their child found that the teen moms who placed their babies for adoption did as well or better than the single teen moms. Those who chose adoption were more likely to complete vocational training, delay marriage, avoid a rapid repeat pregnancy, work after the birth, and be financially better off.

Both groups of teens reported very high levels of satisfaction with their decision. Both groups believed they made the right decision for themselves and their child. Most important, the researchers found that teen moms who placed their child for adoption did not suffer any more negative psychological consequences than the teens who raised their children as single parents.[6]

Why People Adopt Children

Today it's estimated that there are one to two million individuals and couples who want to become adoptive parents. Right now, most parents of adopted infants are infertile couples. They are biologically unable to have a child. There are others who may have already had children, but want to raise another child. There are still other individuals who have always dreamed of having a child and adoption provides them the opportunity to realize this dream. All these people have one thing in common: They want to experience the love and joy which comes from parenting a child.

The following letter was written by an adoptive father to his own mother the day he was united with his adopted son. He and his wife had wanted to have a family for a very long time. You can feel the love and joy this father has for his son.

Dear Mother:

I just can't go to bed tonight without telling you how thrilled and happy Robin and [I] are at this moment. It is eleven years ago today that we were married, and looking back over the years I must say they have been happy, prosperous perhaps, yet they have been saddened by the fact that it seemed inevitable that we were not to be blessed with children. For some time now we have secretly entertained the idea that we would adopt a child, and we are most proud to tell the world that on this, our anniversary, the most beautiful darling boy of six months was brought to us. . . . Robin just brought him in and put him in his crib here for the first time. Mother, the little fellow is a perfect sweet heart.

. . . Mother—we are happy.

Ira

Adoption has its advantages. Even though the acceptability of parenting and abortion has widened the options for teens, the realities of parenting haven't changed. It's just as tough raising a child today, whether you raise your child alone or with the help and support of your boyfriend and/or family. Adoption is a good option for a young woman who is unwilling or unable to have an abortion and who does not want to parent her child. Research has shown that there are tangible benefits for young women who place their infants for adoption. Compared to single teen moms, teens who chose adoption were less likely to be poor, less likely to have received a form of public assistance during the past year, were more likely to have completed more education, and were less likely to become pregnant again soon after the first birth.[7]

It's okay to delay parenting until you are older, have completed your education, and have had more life experiences. Choosing adoption may be the best option for you. It is a responsible decision. In fact, it is a very loving, selfless decision. Choosing adoption provides your child with an opportunity to have a better life than what you could presently provide for him. It also gives an adoptive parent or couple the chance to fulfill a desire to raise a child.

Adoption has its disadvantages. You will experience pregnancy. On the outside you will look pregnant and on the inside you will feel pregnant. This may or may not be a problem for you. If you don't want your friends to know you are pregnant, it can be arranged for you to live and go to school someplace else. This doesn't mean you have anything to be ashamed of, it is merely an option for some young women who may feel uncomfortable being around their peers once they begin to look pregnant. Attending another school temporarily may ease your discomfort.

If you choose to parent your child rather than place your child for adoption, you will experience the hardships which come from early parenting. It will be more difficult for you to complete your schooling, and you will be likely to have financial difficulties which may last until your child is older. You will experience the loss of your youth and freedom. When you choose adoption you end your legal right to parent your child. After experiencing pregnancy for nine months it may be difficult for you to place your child in someone else's care. You will experience a loss, but you can handle this loss with support and counseling. Remember, however, you will experience a loss no matter which option you choose.

Decision-Making Process

Adoption is a deeply personal decision to make. For many women it is not an easy decision to make. Adoption is a legal process which permanently transfers all your parenting rights and responsibilities to an adoptive parent or couple. Once the adoption process is completed it will be very difficult to reverse your decision. It almost never happens. In order for you to regain custody, you will have to prove that the process was done under a great deal of stress or was based on fraudulent information. This is a difficult legal process and one which you should try to avoid.

This isn't meant to scare you. Adoption is the right option for some young women. It's important that you carefully think through this and all of your options. Only you can determine if adoption is best for you at this point in your life. Carefully thinking through the following questions may help you decide if adoption is the best option for you:

Am I able to provide my child with the quality of life I feel she deserves?

Only you know if you are capable right now of being the best parent your child can have. Everyone can be a parent, but not everyone can be a good parent. Not everyone is ready at a certain age to be a good parent. This is the same with other major decisions in your life. You might graduate from high school at age eighteen. But you might not be ready to go on to vocational school or to college. You might turn thirty, but you may still not be ready to marry and have a family. Some women and men feel strongly that they don't ever want to have children; they don't want to be burdened with the responsibility or the lifestyle changes which come with parenting.

Am I willing to make sacrifices in my life in order to raise a child at this time?

When you choose to be a parent there are sacrifices which need to be made. A baby demands a lot of time and energy. This doesn't change much even as a child grows older. There are losses with parenting at a young age.

You lose your freedom. You lose your childhood. Gone are the days when you could just hang out with your friends. Any extra cash you have will be spent on diapers, not lipstick. Of course there is a lot to be gained from being a parent. A child brings a lot of joy into your life. Only you know if the benefits of parenting outweigh the losses in your lifestyle which you will experience at this time.

Can I accept knowing that someone else will permanently parent my child?
    This question gets to the heart of whether or not adoption is the right option for you. When you choose adoption you permanently give your legal right to raise your child to someone else. This means that you and your child will live separate lives. You will not make decisions about your child's life. This is not an issue for some women; it is a loss which they can handle. They go on and live fulfilling lives. For other women it is an issue. It's hard for some women to watch someone else babysit their child; the thought of someone else permanently caring for their child is not something they can accept.

Can I accept that my family or friends may not agree with my adoption plan?
    Your family or friends may not agree with your adoption plans. However, any option you choose may not be accepted by your family or friends. That doesn't mean adoption is a bad decision. Sometimes people whose opinions you value, like your friends and family, may disagree with your decision. This may hurt. It may be helpful to talk to someone who is objective such as a counselor or another adult. They can help you sort out your feelings, and help you when you do talk to people close to you about your adoption plans.
    Adoption is your decision to make. You don't need to justify your decision to anyone. It's no one's business. You don't need your parents' consent. However, the legal process may be confusing. Emotionally you may want their support. In some states you may need your boyfriend's consent. You, your parents, and boyfriend can talk to a counselor. This may help them understand your choice. Counseling may not change their minds, but it's still your decision to make. You need to consider how you will feel if you don't do what you want to do. For example, you may be angry at yourself if you kept your child for your parents and your parents aren't there for you when you need them.

Changing Adoption Practices

Traditionally adoptions have been arranged in a closed, confidential manner. This was done because it was believed to be in the best interest of everyone to protect the privacy of all parties. It protects the identity of the woman who places her baby for adoption, many of whom do not want the circumstances surrounding the birth of their child known. Years ago, young women who placed their babies for adoption were single and ashamed about their pregnancies. A closed adoption allowed them to hide their pregnancy. It allows adoptive parents who may be embarrassed that they are unable to have biological children to keep their child's adoption secret. Some adoptive parents insist on closed adoptions. They fear that their child will experience emotional confusion from having contact with the birth parents.

In a closed adoption the adoptive parents and the birth mother do not know each other's identity. Typically they know nonidentifying information, including medical histories, physical descriptions, and social information. To protect confidentiality in adoption, all records of the adoption process are sealed once the process has been completed. The child's original birth certificate is sealed. A new birth certificate is issued with the child's adopted name and name of the adoptive parents. The original birth certificate and adoption records can be opened only if ordered by the court.

Societal attitudes are changing and adoption practices are now becoming more open. Much of this change has occurred because birth parents, adoptive parents, and adopted children felt it was needed. They felt the old process didn't work. They view closed adoptions as unhealthy and as a way of reinforcing the secrecy and shame which was associated with out-of-wedlock births. Today if a birth mother desires she can still have a closed adoption or she can choose to have an open adoption in which she can have an active role in the adoption process.

"Open adoption" refers to varying degrees of contact with the adoptive parents and possibly the child. It can be confusing, as there is no formal definition of either an open or closed adoption. Each agency has its own practices. In some cases the birth mother can review a list of family profiles and pictures of potential adopters, and pick the individual or couple she feels would provide a good home for her baby. In an even more open adoption she may meet the adopters. In the most open of adoptions, the birth mother has some kind of ongoing contact with the adopters and the child throughout the child's life.

ADOPTION AGENCIES

Adoptions can be arranged through an agency or through an intermediary such as a lawyer. Most, however, are arranged through adoption agencies. There are different types of adoption agencies. There are local- or state-licensed public agencies, and there are private agencies. A public agency is supported by tax dollars; a private agency is supported through fees paid by adoptive families or charitable contributions. Each agency may provide different services. For instance, some agencies may be able to assist you with services you may need, such as prenatal care, and/or temporary housing, and some may not. Some agencies may be able to continue to provide you with services even if you change your mind during your pregnancy and decide you do not want to place your child for adoption. Most adoption specialists recommend women utilize an adoption agency because it offers more protection through state supervision and it offers postadoption counseling and support services.

Adoption laws vary from state to state. For instance, adoptions arranged through a lawyer are not legal in all states. In some states the father of your baby may need to give his consent for the adoption to take place and in other states his consent is not required. Because state laws vary and each agency's practices may differ in what they can provide, it's best for you to ask each agency specific questions, so that you know what to expect. You can locate an adoption agency by looking in the Yellow Pages under "Adoption Agencies."

Adoption Process

Continue to explore the adoption process if you think this option may be best for you. You have time to do this if you are planning to continue your pregnancy. It may help you to meet other teens who have chosen to place their babies for adoption. You might also find it useful to speak to parents who have adopted children. Exploring the adoption process is not a commitment to adoption. Adoption does not become final until after the birth of your child and until you have signed the surrender papers. If you have any lingering doubts about adoption after the birth of your baby, you can postpone the adoption process until you have made up your mind. Although many teens prefer to have their baby placed directly from the hospital with an adoptive family, some teens who aren't quite sure either bring their baby home with them, or place their baby in temporary foster care.

Bringing your child home with you may make your decision a little more difficult because a bond forms between you and the baby, and that bond is strengthened with the amount of time you spend with the child. Some teens do change their minds after bringing their baby home, but some do not. In either case, you will have to deal with a loss. The decision whether to raise your baby is always yours to make. The important thing for you to consider is which option will ensure that the baby will always have someone who will provide loving and constant care. You should never feel pressured, although it's best for both you and your baby if you don't delay your decision for too long.

One young woman, Francine, had difficulty making up her mind. She initially brought her baby home from the hospital, then realized that placing her baby for adoption was the best thing for her to do. Francine explains:

> I thought about adoption all during my pregnancy. I worked with an adoption agency. They were very kind to me. They never pressured me at all. They were very clear with me about my legal rights. They wanted to make sure I made the best decision for myself. All along I had serious doubts about my ability to be a good mother. I was an only child. I was used to being pampered. I had never taken on that kind of responsibility before. I was a cheerleader, and liked hanging out with my friends. My boyfriend said he would help me with our baby, and my parents were also supportive. Their support made my decision harder to make. Because they offered to help me raise my child I felt obligated to be a parent even though I thought adoption would be better. I couldn't decide either way, so I continued to go through the adoption process. I chose the adoptive parents. I even met them. After the delivery of my baby girl, Janine, I decided I'd raise her. Once we got home, I knew I had made the wrong decision. It hurts me to admit it, but I wasn't being a good mother. I fell apart when she cried, and I wasn't able to comfort her. After a couple of weeks, I decided adoption really was best for Janine and myself. Janine was placed with the adoptive parents I had chosen.

Everyone's needs are different. Some teens find it more comforting to have an agency pick their child's parents. Some teens don't feel the need to know the identity of the adoptive parents. They don't have a need for continued contact. It's okay to allow the agency to choose the parents of your child. Adoption agencies carefully select adoptive parents. It's normal to worry and think about how your child is doing.

Sometimes teens choose an open adoption because they are holding on to the hope of a relationship with their child later in life. Sometimes they think it will ease their pain to see their child on a regular basis. Open adoptions are still relatively new. No one knows the long-term effects for everyone involved. *When you choose adoption you give up your legal rights to your child. Open adoption does not give you any legal rights to your child.* Only you know if continued contact with your child will cause you more pain. It may prevent you from getting on with your life.

Because the adoption process varies, it's best to talk to different agencies. Find out what each agency's rules are. Ask questions so you understand their practice. If you feel pressure in any way, talk to another agency. There are many different agencies and you should be able to find one which will meet your needs. Don't go through the adoption process alone. You don't need your parents' permission to place your child for adoption, but it's a good idea to have an adult with you. You can rely on them for emotional support and to help untangle the legal aspects of adoption. Below are some questions which you may want to ask as you talk to different adoption agencies.

QUESTIONS TO ASK

- What are the types of adoptions available to me (closed, open, or a temporary arrangement such as foster care), and what are the pros and cons of each?
- Will there be an opportunity for me to meet with other teens who have chosen adoption, or with an adoptive parent or adoptive couple?
- What role will I have in selecting the adoptive family I would like for my baby?
- How does your agency evaluate potential adoptive couples? How will I know they will be good parents for my child?
- What counseling services are available to me before and after the adoption?
- What are the laws in my state regarding the following: signing the consent forms, revoking consent, finalizing the adoption process, the legal rights of my baby's father, and how the mutual consent birth registry works?

MUTUAL CONSENT REGISTRIES

You may hear people talk about mutual consent registries. These are adoption registries which many states have created to provide a designated place in which both birth parents and adult adoptees can register their names to let it be known that they would like to arrange a meeting. If the parties are interested in meeting, an intermediary will make the necessary arrangements for one to take place. To enroll, you place your name, address, and telephone number with an adoption registry. You can enroll at any time. The information should be kept up to date so that your child will be able to locate you once he or she reaches adulthood.

Many teens think about filing their names with an adoption registry. It may help you to know that your child can look you up if he wants to meet you. Some adoption counselors recommend that you wait before registering with a mutual consent registry because your child can't look you up until he reaches adulthood, and that's a long way off. You may change your mind by then.

Loss Associated with Adoption

There are a lot of emotions involved with adoption which may cause you inner conflict. Deep in your heart you may feel that adoption is the best option for you and your baby. You may be content with your decision. At the same time you may be experiencing a range of other emotions which may cause you some pain. You may be sad when you think of your baby. You may be angry and disappointed in yourself for getting pregnant. You may be angry at your parents or your boyfriend if they are not giving you the support you want. These feelings are all normal. You are not alone. Other young women have experienced these feelings and have found positive ways to manage them.

The loss you experience with adoption is different from the loss you would experience if you had an abortion or if you chose to parent your child. The experience of not parenting your child is a loss and you will go through a mourning period. You will experience pain. This is normal. Any time we experience a loss we feel pain; it is a healthy sign of mourning. Finding positive ways to manage your pain helps to ease it. Adoption is no different from other losses you may have experienced in that the pain you feel can be healed.

Everyone experiences this pain differently. Some women feel very little pain. Some women begin to grieve and mourn their loss during pregnancy and are surprised when they don't feel more pain after the birth of their baby. Other women don't experience their pain until years later. There may be times when you feel more pain. Some teens have found that leaving their baby for the last time, signing the surrender papers, and the baby's first birthday are particularly difficult times. Preparing for these times may not take the pain away, but finding positive ways to cope will help to ease the pain.

Placing your baby for adoption does not mean you stop loving your baby. You may always have maternal feelings for your baby. The love you have for your baby is one of the reasons you made your choice. You may be sad that you will not watch your child grow. This is a loss. However, your loss may be softened knowing you did what was best for you and your baby. You can take comfort knowing that your baby will be raised by loving parents who want a child very much.

Sometimes women have been told that the best remedy for their pain is to "forget about their baby" and "get on with their lives." This isn't a problem for some women. Some women don't dwell on their decision. They have other plans for their life that don't involve raising a child. They want to put off starting a family until they are older. Sometimes women don't want to have a family at all. Other women do experience some pain even though they are comfortable with their decision. You can handle your loss. Accepting that you made the decision and that the decision was best for you and your baby will help to ease your loss. Taking part in the adoption process will also help.

Make your decision freely because it is what *you* want to do. In the long run you will be happier with your decision if you have control in making it. Don't be forced into adoption or any other option. Keep in mind that if you want to place your child for adoption and your family does not support you, there are resources available to you. *To thine own self be true.* Be honest with yourself. Know your limitations. Know your needs. Do what you believe is best for you and your baby.

The feelings you have for your baby and the reasons you chose adoption are unique to you. Allow yourself to experience them. Accept your reasons for choosing adoption. They are right for you. No one else knows the dreams you have for yourself and for your baby, and you are the only one who knows what's best for you and your baby.

SUGGESTIONS FOR COPING WITH LOSS

- Don't be too hard on yourself. Recognize that you made the best decision at this time in your life for both you and your baby.
- Give yourself permission to grieve. Don't deny your feelings. Let the people who are supportive of you know when you're having a tough time.

- Understand that the pain you feel eases with time. As you get on with your life your pain will get better.
- Keep busy. Stay focused on your goals and your education. Take up a hobby. Participate in a sport. Be good to yourself.
- Find a counselor who can help you sort out your emotions. It's important to work with a counselor who understands the grief and the healing processes connected with adoption. Your counselor may help you join a support group that's right for you. It may help you to understand that what you're experiencing is not as uncommon as you think.
- Take part in the adoption process. Your counselor can work with you to help you determine what's important for you to do. Choose an adoption agency that's willing to help you meet your needs. Talk to your health care provider about your feelings. They will help you have the type of birth experience you want. Spend as much time in the hospital with your baby as you want. Take pleasure in bathing, diapering, and feeding your baby. Name your baby. Some teen moms don't want to see their baby. That's okay, but keep in mind that it may be difficult for you to work through your grief if you never allow yourself to see your baby.
- Keep a journal. Sometimes writing can be a great outlet for your pain.
- Develop a strategy for dealing with your emotions on tough days, for example, Mother's Day or your baby's birthday. Recognize that it's normal to remember these days. Take a few minutes to think about your baby and remind yourself why you made your decision.
- Release your pain. Resolve any negative feelings about the adoption which make you feel you did something bad. Write a letter to yourself. Write about all the feelings you are experiencing that are causing you pain. Then burn your letter, bury it, or send it out to sea. Sometimes doing something physical helps you to let go, so that your pain is no longer haunting you.
- Don't sign the surrender papers unless you are absolutely certain about your decision.
- Forgive everyone you feel let you down. Forgive your parents, friends, and/or boyfriend if they did not respond to your pregnancy the way you wanted. Most of all, forgive yourself.

Notes

1. Information on well-known people who have been adopted provided by the National Adoption Information Clearing House, 5640 Nicholson Lane, Suite 300, Rockville, Maryland 20852.

2. S. D. McLaughlin, *Evaluating the Adoption Component of AFL Care Demonstration Projects (Final Report)* (Washington, D.C.: Office of Adolescent Pregnancy Programs, Department of Heath and Human Services, 1991) as cited in the National Council for Adoption, "Fact Sheet on Adoption" (pamphlet) (Washington, D.C.: National Council for Adoption, 1993).

3. M. Custer, "Adoption As an Option for Unmarried Pregnant Teens," *Adolescence* 28, no. 112 (1993): 891–902.

4. Ibid.

5. E. Mech, *Orientation of Pregnancy Counselors toward Adoption (Final Report)* (Washington, D.C.: Office of Adolescent Pregnancy Programs, Department of Health and Human Services, 1984) as cited in E. Mech, "Pregnant Adolescents: Communicating the Adoption Option," *Child Welfare* 65, no. 6 (1986): 555–67.

6. S. D. McLaughlin, D. L. Manninen, and L. D. Winges, "Do Adolescents Who Relinquish Their Children Fare Better or Worse Than Those Who Raise Them?" *Family Planning Perspectives* 20, no. 1 (1988): 25–32.

7. Ibid. and C. A. Bachrach, "Adoption Plans, Adopted Children, and Adoptive Mothers," *Journal of Marriage and the Family* 48 (1986): 243–53.

7

Case Studies:
Raising a Child

In this chapter you will read about two young women, Jennifer and Kate, who raised their babies. They both wanted to be mothers very much, and each looked forward to raising her baby. Jennifer and Kate had already graduated from high school when they gave birth to their babies. Their experiences are somewhat different. Jennifer did not plan to get pregnant; Kate did. Jennifer initially married her boyfriend. Kate never had her boyfriend's or her parents' support. Both felt overwhelmed and isolated at times. Both joined a young parents' support group which helped them. Kate initially had a very tough time. She found parenting to be lonely and exhausting, which she never anticipated. Kate became depressed. She received assistance from a support group for young parents and coped much better, and began to enjoy motherhood.

Jennifer

Jennifer was seventeen years old and a senior in high school when she got pregnant. She didn't use birth control even though she knew about it. She married her boyfriend after becoming pregnant and raised her child alone when the marriage didn't work out. She shares her story so others will know what it's like to be married and raise a child at a young age.

There isn't a quick and easy way to sum up how I felt when I found out I was pregnant. For starters, I got pregnant the first time I had sex, so I really

145

felt unlucky. I felt like the odds were against me. I felt stupid and ashamed because I knew about contraceptives. I remember feeling awkward about my body. I hadn't planned to have sex so I wasn't prepared. My boyfriend and I had never talked about birth control. I also felt trapped because I believed my only option was to get married and raise my child. It never occurred to me that I could raise my child alone. I was brought up to believe that it just wasn't done that way.

My periods were always regular. When I was a few days late, I knew I was pregnant. I told Tom about my fears, and he told me not to worry. He told me right away that he would marry me if that's what I wanted. We went to a clinic and got the news together. We took a long walk through a park and discussed our feelings and how we would tell our parents. I was afraid to tell my parents. I knew they were going to be really upset. I knew I had disappointed them. I knew they would be afraid for me and the fate of my child.

My parents had been through this before with my brother Ron and his girlfriend Judy. Ron and Judy were sophomores in high school when Judy got pregnant. They chose to tell their parents. Judy's mother pressured her to terminate the pregnancy, while my parents encouraged them to raise their baby. They offered emotional and financial support. Ultimately Ron and Judy decided it was best to terminate the pregnancy. I always felt Judy's mother forced her to have an abortion, and their experience had a lot to do with how I felt about abortion. I was not opposed to abortion for religious reasons, it just was not an option for me. Adoption wasn't an option for me either, because I couldn't imagine not knowing my child. I had done a lot of babysitting, and I knew I liked children. I knew I would love my child and do whatever it took to raise her. Getting married and raising my child seemed to me to be the responsible thing to do. I didn't want to disappoint or hurt my parents any more than I already had.

I was graduating from high school and Tom was graduating from college. He already had a job with his family's business. I had no plans to go to college. I hadn't really thought about a career. All I ever wanted was to be a wife and mother, but I didn't want to start this soon and not this way. Tom didn't want me to have an abortion. I was nervous about marrying Tom. We had only been dating for a couple of months. I liked him a lot. We always had fun when we were together. I suppose I was in love, but it's hard to know. We had just started getting serious when I got pregnant. I was scared because it was happening so fast. I guess I was also relieved that he wanted to marry me and take responsibility for a family so soon.

Tom and I told our parents together. Both sets of parents were shocked.

Tom's parents thought we were too young to get married. They suggested I have an abortion or consider adoption. Telling my parents wasn't as bad as I thought it would be. Once they got over their shock they were supportive. I never had my dream wedding. We had a small wedding with just our immediate family. We didn't have a honeymoon; we moved into our own apartment.

My dream of a happy marriage and big family with Tom never came true. My idea of married life was much different from Tom's. I had expectations that we would do things as a family, that Tom would take care of our child and that he would be there for me when I needed him. Tom just wasn't able to do any of these things. I thought it would be better when our baby was born, but it got worse. At first he tried. He went with me to a couple of my prenatal appointments, and to the childbirth classes. He was with me when our daughter, Emily, was born. He seemed so happy. It didn't last long. I remember us arguing a lot, mostly about money. We had agreed I should be home with Emily. When the bills started coming in Tom began complaining. He started working longer hours, then he just stayed out late with the guys. He was never home. Tom felt trapped. He blamed me for ruining his life. He became physically and verbally abusive. I couldn't raise Emily like this, so when she was six months old we separated. We divorced a year later.

After my separation, Emily and I moved in with my parents for almost three years. It was a real struggle to get Tom to pay child support. I got a job right away. I worked in a factory for five dollars an hour. I hated my job. There was no future in it. But it paid the bills and allowed me to be with Emily during the day. My parents babysat for Emily while I worked nights. I saved as much money as I could so I could attend a local community college. I needed to be able to support Emily and myself. I worked part-time and went to school full-time. Eventually I was able to rent a small apartment. It was in a lousy neighborhood, very unsafe, but that was all I could afford. I felt I had made a mistake by getting pregnant and marrying the wrong man. It was up to me to make things right. I was reluctant to ask for help.

There is a lot to think about if you're planning on raising your child. You need to be prepared to raise your child alone. You can't always depend on your boyfriend. Just because your boyfriend sees your baby's birth doesn't mean that he will be there for you. If he is not emotionally ready to be a parent, chances are he won't be there for you or your baby.

Ultimately it is the mother who is responsible for her child. Being responsible means being there for your child twenty-four hours a day. There is a lot to juggle if you have a job and are also going to school. You can't always rely on your family to babysit so you can get a break and go out with your friends. After a while you lose touch with your friends. You have different priorities.

It's tough to raise a child when you're young even if you have good support systems. My daughter turned out well without her father, but every child deserves a father, whether her parents are married or not. It's only natural to want to share the ups and downs of child rearing with your baby's father. If you don't think you can raise your child alone, then I feel you need to think about your other options.

I remember nights when I would cry myself to sleep. I would feel scared and alone. There is so much responsibility, and sometimes it was overwhelming. I didn't have much of a social life. I didn't date for a long time. I didn't have the time. I also didn't feel like I could trust men. I love my daughter; she has brought a lot of happiness into my life. But being single and not having your life together and being responsible for a baby is frightening at times. I finally joined a support group for young moms. It helped talking to other young moms and hearing how they coped.

The experience of becoming pregnant before marriage is still a little painful to me. I wish I had done things the right way. The fact that my marriage was a disaster and my daughter has grown up with limited contact with her father has caused me a great deal of pain. For several years, Emily's father visited her almost every other weekend for a few hours, but he was never there to celebrate her birthdays, school achievements, dance recitals, or any other special events. He wasn't ever there to care for her when she was sick, teach her how to deal with bullies, or to help her with her homework. It's hard to have a parent/child relationship with such limited contact. Emily's father disappeared just before her tenth birthday. He also stopped paying the court-ordered child support.

Tom and I had our baby because we thought we were being responsible. We never talked about what it would be like to be parents. We really didn't know each other. We didn't have the same values. Our relationship wasn't solid enough to survive the hardship of raising a child at a young age. The divorce was very hard on me. It added another stressor for me on top of trying to be a good mother. Who knows if it would have been better to have stayed single and raised Emily on my own. Maybe I wouldn't have had to endure the abuse. Maybe I would have felt able to date sooner. Maybe I would have married sooner and had more children. These are things I'll never know.

When I first became pregnant I was ashamed. I felt very bad when my marriage failed. I am no longer ashamed. I accept that things happen and you deal with them the best you can. My motto has always been that when life gives you lemons, you make lemonade. I refuse to give up. Life does get better if you work hard and believe in yourself.

I have never been sorry that I chose to continue my pregnancy. Emily has helped me to grow up and has given me endless joy. She is the center of my life and the source of my desire to keep going and make a better life.

I finally graduated from college. I finished so that I could get a decent job to support us. I bought a home so that Emily would have security. This time our home is in a nice neighborhood. Eventually it got easier. As I became more serious about achieving my goals people were there to help. I got scholarships to pay for day care from the community college I attended. My parents babysat when I needed to study. My teachers postponed exams if they knew I was out because Emily was sick. I kept plugging away. I didn't want to be a statistic. I wanted to beat the odds.

I have since remarried. I have a wonderful husband and a large family. I married my best friend. We knew each other for a long time before getting involved. Emily has two stepsisters and one stepbrother. My dreams came true. It just took a long time and a lot of determination.

RECAP

Jennifer became pregnant the first time she had sex because she was not using birth control. This has happened to other teens. If you have sex and don't use birth control, the chances of becoming pregnant are very high. Jennifer chose to parent her child because she didn't feel comfortable with her other options. Unlike most teens today, Jennifer and Tom got married. They thought they were ready to be married and raise a child. They thought they were being responsible. Like many teens who get married, their marriage didn't work out. They were divorced before their baby reached her second birthday. Jennifer was very determined to make her life and her child's life better.

FEELINGS

Jennifer experienced a mix of feelings after finding out she was pregnant. She was happy about her pregnancy because she had always dreamed of being a mother, but she was angry and disappointed in herself because she knew about contraceptives and didn't use them. Jennifer was also ashamed about her pregnancy. She wished she had done things differently. She wished she had waited until after she was married before starting a family.

Jennifer was relieved that her parents were supportive of her plans to raise her child. She was hurt and angry with Tom because he was not willing to change his lifestyle and be a parent and husband. She felt bad that her marriage failed and her daughter grew up without a father. Today, Jennifer feels a lot of satisfaction knowing she raised her child on her own despite limited finances and without Tom's support.

REACTIONS

Jennifer didn't waste time feeling sorry for herself when her marriage failed. The loss of her dreams of a happy marriage and family took a back seat to the needs of her daughter. She was very responsible. She sacrificed her own needs in order to care for her daughter. She took a job that she didn't like so she could support herself and Emily. She even delayed her education to do what was best for her child.

COPING

Jennifer relied mostly on her parents for emotional support. She also joined a support group of other young moms. Jennifer was upset when her life didn't work out as she planned, but she remained optimistic and took one step at a time. She knew she had to continue her education so that she could support her daughter. She stayed focused on her goals of completing her education, getting a good job, and securing a safe home for herself and her daughter. She asked for help from her teachers and friends when she needed it.

Kate

Kate was seventeen years old, and a recent high school graduate when she realized she was pregnant. Kate didn't use birth control because she wanted to get pregnant. She was happy about her pregnancy. She chose to raise her baby, even though she didn't have the support of the baby's father or her family.

I was happy when I found out I was pregnant. I've wanted to be a mother since I was a little girl. I had just graduated from high school when I realized I was pregnant. I had a full-time job and was no longer living with my parents. I was able to support both myself and my baby. I was excited about my pregnancy. I was looking forward to being a mother. Having a baby was something I always wanted to do. I felt like I had been given a new beginning to my life. I was very happy. I was in the process of fulfilling a life dream.

In many ways my life was not perfect. Looking back on that time in my life, I realize how alone and isolated I really was. I was so happy about my pregnancy that I didn't stop to take an honest look at my life and to reflect on how a baby would change my life. For the most part, I kept my pregnancy a secret. I didn't tell my family that I was pregnant. I didn't have any close friends to share my pregnancy with. It was easy to hide my pregnancy because I was heavy. I just looked like I had put on a little more weight. Only the people I worked with knew about my pregnancy. I had to tell them so I could arrange for my maternity leave. Because I didn't share my pregnancy with anyone, I had no one I could rely on to discuss my feelings with or to help me plan ahead for the baby. I did everything by myself. Later I realized what a big burden I had taken on. I paid a price for that. I ended up depressed and physically exhausted.

I was sharing an apartment with a friend who was a few years older than me. She was someone I admired and looked up to. She was pretty and had a boyfriend and a great job. She seemed to have her life together. I thought of her as a close friend, but she wasn't really. She was someone who took advantage of me. I couldn't count on her. Eventually she lost her job and broke up with her boyfriend. I ended up paying all the rent and buying her groceries. Instead of being supportive, she added a lot of stress to my life.

I couldn't count on my baby's father or my parents for help and support. My boyfriend, Dave, and I had already broken up by the time I found out I was pregnant. We got together right before graduation and had one last fling. To be honest, I knew about birth control. I had been on the pill. When Dave and I broke up, I went off the pill. The night that Dave and I got together I purposely didn't tell him that I had stopped taking the pill. He didn't seem concerned about it. He never asked about birth control. Besides, I was hoping to get pregnant. I really wanted a baby. I was very happy later when I realized I was pregnant.

I didn't tell Dave I was pregnant until our baby was born. I didn't know how he would react. I was afraid he would try and pressure me into having an abortion. Since we weren't going together anymore, I didn't feel he should have any say about what I chose to do. I have always been opposed to abortion for moral reasons and I wasn't about to have one. I wanted to be a mother. I wasn't going to place our baby for adoption. I also secretly hoped that once he saw his baby, he would want to get back together again.

I couldn't really count on my parents either. I maintained very little contact with them during my pregnancy. They were never supportive of me while I was growing up. I didn't know how they would react, so I kept my pregnancy a secret from them. I had already made up my mind to raise my baby. I didn't want their opinion and I didn't want them to try to change my mind.

I had a miserable childhood. I never felt loved by my parents. They always picked on me. They'd laugh at me and make jokes about me. My mom would complain that I was overweight. It seemed like whatever I did, it was never good enough for them. I was a good student. I had a decent job and was supporting myself, but that wasn't good enough. They'd always find something wrong with me. I never felt accepted by them. It always came back to the fact that they didn't like the way I looked. They couldn't handle the fact that I was overweight.

My parents wanted me to go to college. I figured at some point I'd go to school to be a legal assistant. I had absolutely no intentions of going to college. I wanted to be a mother. I already had a part-time job in a law office, with the promise of full-time employment after graduation. My parents told me without a college degree I'd be a failure, I'd never get anywhere in my life. That was the last struggle we got into. After that I moved away. I couldn't take their criticism anymore.

I told myself that when I was a mother, I'd do things differently. I'd be a really good mom. My child would be my top priority. I would love my child unconditionally. My child would always know she was special and loved from the moment she was born. My life started taking on a new meaning from the moment I found out that I was pregnant. I felt I had a sense of direction and purpose. I finally had someone to love and to love me back. I was eager to prove to my parents that I could be a better parent, that I was independent and responsible.

I actually felt great during my pregnancy. Having a baby was something I really wanted to do, so I got regular prenatal care. I took especially good care of myself during my pregnancy. I had a lot of energy. I worked full-time and sometimes worked overtime so I could save for the baby. I was prepared for the baby. I bought everything ahead of time. Someone from work had already had a baby. She wasn't planning on having anymore children, so she gave me a lot of things.

I started feeling lonely during the last month of my pregnancy. My midwife wanted me to go to childbirth classes. I didn't have anyone I could take with me, so I didn't go. I was sad when I realized I wouldn't have anyone with me during labor. I finally broke down and told my roommate that I was pregnant a couple of weeks before I was due. I was relieved to finally tell her. I was exhausted from trying to hide my pregnancy. I wanted her to be happy for me, but she was angry. She didn't want a baby keeping her up late at night. All she could think about was how a baby would inconvenience her life. She refused to be my labor coach. I felt rejected by her. That's when I realized I had no one I could rely on. I refused to tell my parents. I didn't want them to know until after I delivered my baby.

I had a wonderful childbirth experience. My daughter, Jessica, was a joy to care for from the moment I gave birth to her. She is such a delight, a very good baby. I don't know what I would have done if she were a difficult baby, because my energy level dropped soon after I came home from the hospital. It got worse each day. I was in a deep depression by the time I went for my six-week check-up. I don't know if it was brought on by a touch of the post-partum blues* or because I was isolated and was caring for Jessica all by myself. All of a sudden I really had a hard time getting it together. I didn't want to get out of bed in the morning. Opening a can of formula was a real effort. I had no energy or desire to be around other people. It was a project just to get Jessica ready to go to the grocery store. I couldn't afford a babysitter, so I couldn't ever get a break from caring for Jessica. I felt like all I did was feed, burp, and change my baby every two hours. I was emotionally and physically exhausted. I never planned on feeling this way. I had thought my baby would give me love back, but she didn't. Instead, she demanded constant attention from me.

The way everyone reacted to my baby didn't help my emotional state either. My roommate gave me trouble from the moment I told her about my pregnancy. I thought she would be more supportive once she saw Jessica, but she wasn't. She absolutely refused to help me out with her. She wouldn't even watch her while I took a shower. She had just lost her job, and was having problems with her boyfriend, so she was always hanging around the house watching TV. I felt guilty about my baby. I had a hard time speaking up for myself. She knew that, and took advantage of me. She stopped paying rent. I was afraid we would get evicted. I had no place else to go, so I paid her share of the rent. She wouldn't contribute for groceries either. She kept complaining she didn't have any money. I felt sorry for her and I didn't want to be alone, so I put up with it.

---

*Post-partum blues refers to a feeling of sadness which occurs in about 50–70 percent of new mothers in the days following delivery. These feelings are brought about in part due to the changing hormone levels of your body as it adjusts to no longer being pregnant. Post-partum blues which persist may signal post-partum depression which is serious and should be reported to your health care provider.

My parents were very upset when they found out about Jessica. My dad called me all sorts of bad names. My mom accused me of purposely being mean to her by making her look bad. They both told me I had disgraced them by having a baby out of wedlock. They made it clear that they would not help me out. I felt devastated and let down by what they said. I had this fantasy that they would accept what I had done and love my baby once they saw her. The reality was that they had nothing nice to say to me. They didn't think I was being responsible at all. They told me what I had done was very irresponsible. Once again, I felt like I could never measure up to their expectations of me. As usual I felt rejected by my parents. I never anticipated my parents' reactions. I was hoping my parents would take an active part in Jessica's life. I was very hurt by the things they said.

Dave was shocked when I called to tell him about Jessica. At first he refused to acknowledge that he was her father. He accused me of falsely naming him as the father. When I reminded him of our last fling he reluctantly agreed that he could be the father. He yelled at me. He was furious at me for not telling him that I had gone off the pill. He said I had deceived him and I deserved whatever happened to me. He told me I had no right to look for support from him, since he felt I would never have gotten pregnant in the first place if I had been honest with him about being off the pill. He absolutely refused to see Jessica. That night I cried myself to sleep. Dave's reaction left me feeling sad, rejected, unloved, and totally alone.

I never fully anticipated Dave's reactions. I had such a strong desire to be a mother and have a family that I thought Dave would come around. I was devastated by his lack of interest in me and Jessica. At first I refused to accept that he didn't want to see us. From time to time, I would walk by where he worked with Jessica to try to bump into him, but I never did. I kept thinking he would change his mind once he saw how beautiful she was. Once in a while he sends money. But it's not that much. I know he made it clear to me that he wants nothing to do with us, but I still hope he changes his mind.

I was very unhappy and depressed when I went for my six-week postpartum check-up. My midwife kept asking me a lot of questions. She sensed there was something wrong with me by the way I looked and acted. Finally I broke down and cried. I must have cried for an eternity. She sat there and listened to everything I said. She told me she was concerned about me. She thought I needed some emotional support. This scared me, because I've never been used to relying on others for help or emotional support.

She referred me to a young mothers' support group. At first, I wasn't really interested in the support group. I had to go back to work in two weeks. I didn't know how I would find the time or energy to go to the meetings. I couldn't see what I was going to get out of it. I thought it would be a real hassle, but it turned out to be just what I needed.

My midwife made the first call for me while I was in her office. After my appointment, I met with the coordinator of the support group. At first I was very distrustful. I just kind of listened to what people said. I kind of just went along with everything. I was afraid that if I didn't they'd take Jessica away from me. I find it very hard to trust people. Other than my midwife, no one has ever taken an interest in me before. My parents were always telling me that I was a failure. I remember wondering why anyone would want to help me. Eventually I started to trust the people I met in the group and became more active with the group.

I got lots of services from the support group. I met other young mothers who were experiencing a lot of what I was going through. I found a lot of comfort in that. I made some new friends. I was able to get out more with the other young women I met. They had transportation to meetings and special events. Once in a while just the moms would go out. They provided a babysitter for us on these special occasions. For the first time in a long time I did not feel as isolated. I began to feel cared about and accepted as a person. I also felt better about how I was caring for Jessica. I felt a lot better about myself.

I got matched with a parenting mentor named Peg who was the mother of two toddlers. She spent a lot of time with me. She'd meet me at my house or on nice days we'd meet at a playground. She gave me a lot of positive support. She reminded me of all the good things I was doing. She was always there for me. She nurtured me. She gave me a lot of attention and emotional support. She also taught me how to care for Jessica. There was a lot about being a mother that I just had no clue about. She gave me great advice. She really helped me out the most. Without her kindness, patience, and guidance I don't know how I would have made out. It scares me to think that things might have gotten worse.

She helped me sign up for WIC.* I didn't realize how expensive it was to raise a child. I didn't count on missing days from work because my baby was sick. She also gave me some ideas on how to deal with my roommate. I had never been assertive before. I was always the kind of person that

---

*Recall that WIC is a program which provides nutritious food to eligible women, infants, and children.

people walked all over and took advantage of. Once I started feeling better about myself I was able to assert myself with my roommate. For the time being, we have a better relationship now. She's paying her share of the rent and is slowly paying me back the money she owes me. She's moving out in a couple of months. I made friends with someone in my parent group. She's going to move in with her son. This is a better arrangement for everyone.

Jessica just turned a year old. It's still a struggle. There are days when I'm very exhausted and wonder how I'm going to get by. But generally, I feel a lot better about myself. I feel I'm the kind of mother I should be and always wanted to be. My baby has also benefitted from the extra attention I got. Jessica's more alert. She's a very happy child. Looking back, I realized I wasn't getting any joy from being a mother. I got no satisfaction from parenting. I had unrealistic expectations of what it took to be a mother and what your baby gives in return.

I know I have a long road ahead of me. My parents and Dave are still not speaking to me. But I've made friends. This is something new for me. Most important, I learned I can count on myself. I am responsible. I am a good mother. I'm doing okay.

RECAP

Kate became pregnant when she didn't use birth control. She wanted to get pregnant; part of her life dream was to be a mother. She had just graduated from high school, had her own apartment, and had a job, so she was able to support both herself and her baby. Kate underestimated how demanding motherhood can be. She did not have any emotional support. She had no one on whom she could rely. She never anticipated that her parents and her baby's father would disapprove of what she had done. Because Kate had few relationships, she didn't have a good sense as to how people would respond. Kate lacked judgment as to how the decisions she made would affect other people. She had unrealistic expectations. She became depressed soon after she gave birth to her baby. She was determined to be a good mother, so when her midwife referred her to a teen mothers' support group she went and was able to receive the assistance and encouragement she needed.

FEELINGS

Kate was very happy and excited about her pregnancy. She had always wanted to be a mother and was glad that she was in the process of fulfilling a life dream. Kate felt rejected by the people she loved and cared about. She had a turbulent relationship with her parents and felt unloved and unaccepted by them. She moved out of their house before she graduated from high school. She had hoped that her parents, old boyfriend, and roommate would be supportive of her pregnancy, but they all reacted negatively. She didn't think about how they would react and wasn't prepared for a negative response. She was very hurt by their response and lack of involvement.

REACTIONS

Kate hid her pregnancy from almost everyone. She had made up her mind about what she was going to do. She was afraid that other people would pressure her to do something that she didn't want to do. Kate became depressed within a short time of her delivery. She was emotionally and physically exhausted and barely able to care for herself and her baby.

COPING

Initially Kate tried to manage everything by herself. She took the entire burden of parenting on herself, but it became too much for her. She confided in her midwife, who referred her to a support program for young mothers. Kate was matched with a parenting mentor who was an older, experienced mother. Kate relied on her parenting mentor for emotional support and guidance with parenting. Kate also met other young moms with whom she became friends. They were a good source of support for her, as she didn't have any friends and she found comfort knowing other young women who were going through similar experiences. She has plans to live with someone from her support group.

8

Case Studies:
Choosing Abortion

꧁•❀•꧂

In this chapter you will read about two young women, Alison and Courtney, who both became pregnant at a time in their lives when they didn't want to. They both chose to terminate their pregnancies. The way they went about making their decision and how they felt about their decision afterward was very different. Alison was much younger than Courtney. She consulted others during her decision-making process. Today she feels comfortable with her decision. Courtney was older and in college at the time of her pregnancy. She made her decision alone. She doesn't feel she had all the facts to make a well-informed decision. She wishes she had thought through her decision more and that she had involved another older, responsible adult with her decision-making process. She has since struggled emotionally with what she did. Today she still wonders if she made the right decision.

Alison

> Alison became pregnant when she was fourteen years old. She knew about birth control but didn't use it, and she was not the first young woman in her class to become pregnant.

I was fourteen when I got pregnant. I knew all about birth control. I knew other kids in my class who had dropped out of school because they were pregnant. I just didn't bother to take any precautions. I figured I was too young to get pregnant. I wasn't like any of the "other girls" in my class who were always getting themselves into trouble. I had an older boyfriend. Because he was older, I figured he was wiser and would protect me from getting pregnant. I didn't get pregnant right away. That's another reason why I took so many chances. I really thought it couldn't happen to me. So each and every time we had sex I was willing to take a chance. My boyfriend never brought up birth control. If he wasn't worried about it, I figured I didn't need to worry about it. We had sex quite a few times before I actually got pregnant. Wow, was I shocked.

John was my boyfriend. Well, I considered him my boyfriend. I'm not really sure how he felt about me. When I found out I was pregnant he certainly backed away very quickly. I was crazy about him. I had liked John for as long as I can remember. I had a lot of feelings about him, more than just a crush. He was the first guy I ever liked. John was seventeen. He was my brother's best friend. He was so different from the other guys I hung around with. He was very good looking. He was big, muscular, very rugged, and athletic. I really liked that. All the guys my age were geeky. I just wasn't attracted to them. I thought they were childish and immature. Because John was my brother's friend we always spent a lot of time together. Usually my brother was around. Once I turned fourteen John used to find reasons to get together with me when my brother wasn't around. He had a car. He used to pick me up after school and take me places. He flirted with me a lot in front of my girlfriends. I was taken in by that. I felt very special.

Fourteen was the year in my life when everything started happening. I suddenly became aware of all these feelings and I had a hard time trying to control them. I wanted to learn as much about life as I could. I loved music. I loved hanging out with my friends. I loved being with John. I liked how I felt when we spent time together. I really wanted to find out what sex was all about. I really wanted to have sex with John. The first time I had sex with John it was just to experiment. Then other opportunities came up, so I continued to have sex with him. There was all this stuff going on in my life that I didn't want to think about, so I guess I used sex to have a good time and block out everything in my life that I didn't want to deal with. Sex wasn't always fun, and it wasn't always great.

My parents had gotten divorced the year before. They weren't happy for quite a while. It took them a long time before they ended their marriage. Even after the divorce they were bitter and angry at each other. My dad got custody of my brother and me. We moved into a new house and I had to switch schools. My mom was just not there for me. She kind of abandoned us, like she just wasn't interested in being a mother or a parent anymore. After my parents' divorce she pulled away from us. I didn't have anyone I could talk to about my feelings. I couldn't talk to my mom. I didn't have an older sister. None of my girlfriends was having sex yet. They didn't know anything or even seem to be interested in finding out about it. So it wasn't like I could talk to them. Who was I supposed to talk to, my dad, my brother? Everything I was feeling then was too personal to share with them. One time I did try to talk to my mom. I told her there was this older guy I liked, that he used to put his arm around me and that I really liked that. She freaked. She couldn't handle it. She's Baptist and spends all day Sunday in church. She told me that I shouldn't be dating any guys, especially older guys. She also told me I would have to deal with my father, because she absolutely would not help me out if I got pregnant. That was our one discussion about sex. There was no "this is normal" to have these feelings at your age, or "this is what the 'birds and the bees' is all about." She jumped to conclusions very quickly. She assumed after a few innocent hugs I would get pregnant. I remember being annoyed with her attitude, but that's sort of what happened.

I instinctively knew I was pregnant the day I didn't get my period when I was supposed to. Unlike a lot of other girls, my periods were always normal. When another two weeks went by, and I still hadn't gotten my period, a real sick, nervous feeling sank in. Each passing day that I didn't get my period, I felt worse and worse. I was stunned. I remember I kept thinking to myself, No way, this can't be happening to me. I waited about three more weeks before doing anything. Then I went alone to a family planning clinic, and got a pregnancy test. I was feeling pretty scared and panicky when I got the results. I told John first. We were about three months into our relationship when I got pregnant. He was not emotional about it. He wasn't interested in being a father at this point in his life. He was very up front and direct about telling me that. He just told me I would have to have an abortion. We never got a chance to talk about it. After that, John definitely avoided me. I felt abandoned by him. I was really hurt. He just dumped me. No explanations. No responsibility. No understanding for me and what I was going through being pregnant.

I didn't know who to turn to. I didn't want to bother my dad. He had been through a lot with my mom and their divorce. He's an important business man, and puts in a lot of hours. Finally, not knowing what to do, but knowing that I needed to talk to someone, I turned to my brother. We were fairly close, and usually shared our problems. My brother was furious with John. He started a big fight. It was awful. I was counting on my brother to help me out. I especially did not want him to talk to my dad about it. I thought he would help me arrange an abortion, but he wouldn't do that. He insisted that I talk with my dad before I did anything. I was afraid to tell my dad. It's not easy talking about sex to your father, especially when you've never talked about that kind of stuff before and you have to drop the news on him that you're pregnant. My brother and I talked about what I should say to my dad. My dad had a lot going on at work and he was working a lot of late-night hours. I didn't want to tell him at work, so I had to stay up late one night. I told him I was pregnant after he put in about a twelve-hour day at work. It wasn't exactly the best timing, but at that point I was desperate and had to tell someone.

Once my dad got over his initial reaction, he was fine. He took off from work the next day, right in the middle of a major deadline for him. He took me to our doctor. He stayed in the waiting room while my doctor examined me. After the exam we talked together with my doctor about what my options were. Adoption was only briefly mentioned. We mostly talked about how my life would change if I had a baby. We talked about what an abortion was and where I could have one if that's what I wanted. My dad never pressured me to have an abortion. He told me he would hire someone to stay with the baby so that I could go back to school. My dad's religious. He didn't believe in abortion, but he didn't object to my having an abortion. He wanted to make sure that I felt comfortable no matter what I did.

I actually tried talking to my mom about what I should do. I guess you could say that was bold of me, considering I already knew how she felt about sex. My mom wouldn't have anything to do with me. She absolutely would not help me out. She would not offer me any advice. She told me to talk to my dad and decide what I wanted to do. My mom is so religious, I think she believed I deserved to get pregnant because I was having sex before being married. We had never had a very good mother-daughter relationship, and my pregnancy strained our relationship even more. The fact that she was not there for me when I needed her really hurt. I've since forgiven my mom, but it's taken many years for us to get closer. I now know and understand my mom much better. I understand now why she wasn't able to help me. She was devastated by my pregnancy. She was brought up not to have premarital sex. It's against her religion, and that belief affected how she reacted to me and my pregnancy.

No one else helped me with my decision. I decided to have an abortion. It took me a couple of weeks to decide. Once I made up my mind I felt very relieved. I was fourteen. I considered myself much too young to be a mother, and much too young to get married. Besides, John did not have the same feelings for me that I had for him. It's not like we could have stayed together and raised our child together. He wasn't willing to be a father at that point in his life. It wouldn't have been impossible for me to care for my baby while I was in school. Some of the other girls in my class did. My father was willing to get me a babysitter, but bottom line, I knew I just wasn't ready to be a mother. Emotionally I didn't have it in me to be a mother at that age. There were so many other things going on in my life. My mom and dad's divorce bothered me. My mom was cold and distant. She wasn't going to help me out. I didn't have any role models. I didn't have any sisters or aunts. I didn't think a babysitter was going to give me the kind of help I needed. I didn't know how to be a mother. Also, I was a decent student. I got all As and Bs. I was already thinking about which college I wanted to attend and what I wanted to study. I knew it wouldn't be impossible for me to raise my baby, because others were doing it. I just knew it wasn't what I wanted to do. Having a baby at age fourteen was not the way I always dreamed my life would turn out. I planned to go to college first, get married, then have kids. You know, do everything the right way.

I had mixed feelings about my abortion. Even though I was relieved after I made my decision, I also felt sad about what I was doing. I never got overwhelmed by my feelings. I didn't dwell on what I had done. That probably helped me cope better.

My dad went with me when I had my abortion. He stayed in the waiting room. I will never forget the fact that my father was there for me, and made sure that I was well taken care of. I will always be grateful that he didn't pressure me. He wasn't happy about my pregnancy or the abortion, but he put his feelings aside to make sure I was okay. My dad also paid for the abortion. I was embarrassed that my dad had to pay for it, but there was no way I could have done it.

My life changed after the abortion. I started hanging out with my girlfriends again. I took a photography class. I bought myself a decent camera and became the class photographer for our yearbook. I didn't get involved with anyone again until I was in college. I also took more responsibility with birth control. I talked to my boyfriend about it, and we both decided together what we would do. I was emotionally stronger then and felt more able to do that. I also knew the consequences and knew I never wanted to have another abortion.

I do not have any regrets about my decision to have an abortion. I couldn't have had a baby then. I think it would have been very irresponsible of me. I wasn't emotionally ready to be a mother. My baby would not have had a father. Even though my dad was willing to help out, I felt I couldn't handle motherhood at that time.

My abortion was not a big loss to me. I was sad that I had to have an abortion. But it was my decision and no one forced me into it. Sometimes I look back and wonder what my life would have been like if I had had my baby. After the abortion I had bad dreams for a while, but I don't have them anymore. I am convinced that I made the right decision for myself at that time in my life. I didn't consider adoption. No one ever really discussed that possibility with me. I'm not going to second guess myself and wonder if that's what I should have done. I'm comfortable with what I did.

RECAP

Alison's experience is similar to that of many other young women. Many young women have become pregnant because they thought like Alison did that "it could never happen to me." Alison terminated her pregnancy. She involved her dad with her decision-making process, but ultimately she made the decision herself. Sometimes she had sad feelings about her decision, but she has no regrets about what she chose to do. She feels she made the best decision for herself at that time in her life.

FEELINGS

Alison felt stunned more than anything else about her pregnancy. She was scared to tell her mother, knowing that she was religious and would not approve of her decision. She was afraid to tell her dad, because she had never talked to him before about sensitive issues and was worried he was too busy to help her out. She found out that her dad was glad she came to him. She was hurt by the way her mother and her boyfriend reacted to her pregnancy. She wanted her mother's help in making her decision. She was angry when her mother distanced herself and wouldn't help her. She wasn't prepared for her boyfriend's reaction. She felt abandoned by him.

REACTIONS

Alison was mostly relieved after her abortion. She was also sad, but she was comfortable with her decision. She had bad dreams for a while. She wonders from time to time what her life would have been like if she had her baby, but she knows what she did was right for her.

COPING

Alison relied on her father for both emotional and financial support for her abortion. After her abortion, she took up a hobby and excelled at it. She became the class photographer. She lost interest in dating for a while. She waited until she was in college before she started dating again. She learned about birth control. She was able to talk to her boyfriend about it and they were both responsible about using birth control.

Courtney

Courtney was twenty years old, just a couple months shy of her twenty-first birthday and in her fourth year of college when she became pregnant. She decided to have an abortion. Her relationship with her boyfriend, which hadn't been going well, ended after she had her abortion. She became pregnant again less than a year later and had another abortion. She decided to share her experience in order to help other young women in similar circumstances with their decision-making process.

I'll begin with Steve. Steve was my first real boyfriend. We met while I was going to college. I was living with a roommate in an off-campus apartment and he was working odd-jobs having already dropped out of a different college. One New Year's Eve a group of friends and I decided to "crash" a party. As I walked through the front door, right at midnight, I happened to notice Steve standing near the entranceway drinking a beer. He was my type of guy, wearing jeans and a flannel shirt, with long, dark hair. As hokey and shallow as this sounds, I fell "head over heels" in love with him. Although I had had other boyfriends, I had not yet been "in love."

Later on we had sexual intercourse. It was my first time, but it wasn't Steve's. Even though he was not a virgin, we were both quite naive about sex, and in particular the use of birth control. We used no protection. Unfortunately, I got pregnant the very first time I had sex.

Missing a period was foreign to me. I always had a regular cycle. However, I instinctively knew I was pregnant when I did not have my period on the date it was due, and when I began to experience intense and frequent nausea. I still waited two more weeks before scheduling a pregnancy test at a community clinic. I'm not sure why I waited.

I felt miserable during that time. I felt alone, afraid, and overwhelmed. I was probably in shock. I was on automatic pilot. My actions were robotlike. I went to work and went to classes. I did everything that I would normally do. When I think back about it, I'm amazed that I was able to handle my responsibilities while at the same time trying to cope with such acute feelings of panic, isolation, and fear.

I was much different then than I am now. Back then, I was a very private person, almost pathologically so. I found it tremendously difficult to discuss my situation with anyone other than Steve. Don't get me wrong, Steve and I were not emotionally intimate, then or ever. We never had a meaningful or mature discussion about the pregnancy or our feelings for each other. However, there was no one else I could turn to. I wasn't close to my family, and so I didn't feel I could turn to my parents or any of my brothers and sisters for support. I was also hesitant to turn to my friends. My friends, as I look back, were more social friends. They were not friends I could trust. They were not friends I felt I could bare my soul to. I had no soul mate.

I remember being too afraid to go alone to get the pregnancy test. Steve was unable, or unwilling, to go with me to the clinic. I'm not sure where Steve was at that time or why he couldn't go with me to the clinic. Whatever the reason, he wasn't there for me. I know by that time I had told him that I thought I was pregnant. I was becoming increasingly disappointed in him. I wanted him to be more involved with my situation and more supportive.

Even though I would have preferred Steve's company if he was available, I had decided to confide in a friend, Beth, about my situation. I asked her to go with me to the clinic. Beth was one of the group of friends that had gone to the New Year's Eve party with me and she knew Steve. She was also a student at the college and happened to work at the campus health center. I counted on her to be understanding and supportive. Needless to say, I pressed her to keep my pregnancy confidential. I made her promise not to tell anyone. At the very least, I did not want to have to go alone to the clinic and I was relieved that Beth was willing to go with me.

However, on the morning of my appointment, Beth was a no-show. She did not meet me as we had planned. I did try to reach her at her dorm, but someone told me that she had spent the night with her boyfriend. I was unable to find her. After all the time I spent planning, I ended up going alone to get the pregnancy test.

That day was a miserable day. I felt betrayed by my "close" friend, Beth. That hurt a lot. Besides all my other concerns and feelings, I was suffering the loss of a good friend. I felt she could give me no explanation (and Beth never gave me one anyway) which would be sufficient to repair the damage done to our friendship.

Maybe I was too hard on Beth and blamed her unnecessarily. I was feeling a lot of pain and anguish then. I was feeling angry at myself for getting pregnant and angry at Steve for bailing out on me. It could be that I took all the pain I was feeling out on Beth. I can say that I never trusted her again. For a very long time I felt nothing but bitterness and anger toward her for bailing out on me.

And what about my feelings toward Steve? He too betrayed me that day. For a long while, I focused my anger only on Beth and seemed to excuse Steve. But the truth was, simply, that he was not in love with me. His attraction to me was mostly physical. This hurt, because I was in love with him. Also, it felt to me during this time that he too bailed out on me.

I have no memory of the actual clinic where I got the test, or the time it took to get the test results back. I do not recall where I was when I was told I was pregnant. And, I do not recall the details of any conversation with the personnel at the clinic. Perhaps my lack of memory is noteworthy. I guess blocking reality was my only way to cope.

I do remember somewhat our brief and strained discussion the night I told Steve I was pregnant. We were at my apartment. We were both still stunned. We were both struggling with my pregnancy, even though one would think we should have known of the risks of having unprotected sex. At some point, Steve asked me if I thought we should get married. There was no excitement. There was no sense of desire that we really wanted to get married. It didn't feel even like we were prepared to get married. Marriage only seemed like a sense of obligation, something that we had to do. "No" was my clear answer to Steve. I was quite sure I did not want to marry him. I had already made up my mind. I had decided to have an abortion. We never even considered adoption during the decision-making process. I also understood that it was my responsibility to arrange the abortion, although I don't remember how we decided that.

During this brief decision-making process, neither one of us sought out guidance from a counselor, priest, parent, or any other older, wiser adult. I'm older now, and I understand the value of involving more knowledgeable people when I make important decisions. As a result of not talking to anyone other than Steve, I never fully considered all my options. I made a decision at a time when I felt panic and fear, and I will always question whether my decision was sound and reasonable.

I believe the only real option I could have considered other than abortion would have been to place my baby for adoption. By then I am sure I realized that Steve would not be a dependable husband or father. I just wasn't comfortable with the idea of getting married to him.

I really did not understand what an abortion was. At that time, I thought it was a form of birth control. I didn't know that an abortion involved the intentional killing of a life. I don't mean that to sound too harsh or judgmental, but that's the fact. It was years later, when I saw a picture of a six-week-old fetus, that I started to absorb the seriousness of my decision.

These are the factors in my decision-making process that I remember being aware of: (1) I was afraid of my parents' reaction and I didn't want to have to tell them of my pregnancy; (2) I knew my parents expected me to finish college, although I also knew that, being Catholic, they would expect me to marry; (3) I wanted to have a career, as well as finish college; (4) I was not ready emotionally or financially to raise a child or to get married. Even though I was in love with Steve, despite his limitations, it did not feel like I was ready for marriage; (5) I felt my friends would abandon me because I was careless and stupid enough to allow myself to become pregnant (most of my friends from college wanted careers); (6) I would have been ashamed to be a single, pregnant girl—at that time, it was still taboo for an upper-middle-class girl to be in such a predicament and I couldn't even comprehend living out that scenario; and (7) I did grow to realize that Steve was an unreliable boyfriend and as a mate, I would be unable to depend on him to take care of me, much less a family. So for all these reasons I chose to have an abortion.

Steve and my roommate, Meg, in whom I had, by that time, confided as well, took me to the clinic to have the abortion. It was a different clinic than the one where I had had my pregnancy test. The building was big, gray, and ugly outside, and the elevator inside was cramped and old. I felt very uncomfortable as I entered the clinic. I felt afraid and ashamed. I remember wanting to ask someone if I could still have children later, when I was ready, but I never did.

Except for sitting in a big chair, among several other women who also had just had abortions, all I remember was paying for the abortion afterward. I have no other memories of the abortion. I just remember that Steve drove Meg and me to a drugstore to buy supplies: sanitary pads, which I had never used before, and aspirin. The clinic didn't provide such items. It's amazing to me, given all I don't remember, that I remember these other details. Steve bought me a couple gifts, a record album (*The Best of the Lovin' Spoonful*) and a couple little bathtub toys. They weren't much comfort because I couldn't take baths for a while. Steve made me lunch back at the apartment, and then left. I was alone again. Meg wasn't really a friend so much as someone to help coordinate driving and errand-running.

Steve dropped out of sight for several months after the abortion. When he finally reappeared, it was only to give me money, repayment for the cost of the abortion. I think it was about $160 in cash. He told me he felt it was his obligation to pay although I had never asked him for the money. We did not talk about the abortion, much less our relationship, anymore. I was devastated that he was so emotionally distant. Although he never directly said this to me, he ended up breaking off our "relationship."

I didn't see Steve again for about a year. The summer after I had the abortion I went to California. I called Steve from there because I wanted to see him again. I asked him to pick me up at the airport when I returned and he agreed. When we got to my parents' house (by then I had moved back in with them) we had unprotected sex. This time I had calculated the days my period would be due, in other words, I tried to follow the rhythm method. When Steve asked me if it would be safe to have unprotected sex, and this time he clearly did ask, I told him that I was due for a period. I made the decision for both of us that it was safe not to use any other form of birth control. I got pregnant a second time.

By then, of course, I was not naive about sex, or protection, or the risks of pregnancy. And when I learned I was pregnant, I merely did what I knew I had to do, what I had done before. I had a second abortion. There was no real thought process involved. I don't recall what I felt. I did tell Steve that I was pregnant again, but Steve told me that he held me fully responsible for the pregnancy this second time, and would not "support" me in any way. We clearly were not boyfriend/girlfriend then. This sexual encounter was a one-night stand kind of thing.

I'm not trying to cop out, but that's all I remember. I know that I agreed with Steve. I also felt responsible for the pregnancy and that he was justified in wanting out of the process. I'm aware of my actions. I actually used sex to re-engage him in a relationship. I acted irresponsibly by not using birth control. I got pregnant and we never got back together again. The wiser thing to do would have been to insist upon using birth control.

Well, what I can say at this point is that writing about this has been extremely difficult. I have not resolved my feelings about these abortions and perhaps never really will resolve them. Anyone reading this should know that I have had years of therapy trying to deal with the pain, shame, guilt, and confusion I feel about my abortions. I am thirty-eight, single, and childless.

Something positive has come from this experience. Since my college years I have learned to fight my tendency to be private and self-contained. I have become a rather open and forthright individual. This is a big change for me, a good change for me. I no longer isolate myself. I am able to express as well as share my feelings with other people. I am much more confident in myself. There is of course one exception. I do not discuss this painful subject with everyone. I'm not ready to do that. I share my experience now so that others in the same situation will benefit from what I learned.

I have a successful career. In fact, I am a lawyer and I concentrate in the representation of children, mostly abused and neglected children. Sometimes I wonder if I'm doing this as a way of redeeming myself. I don't know. Even though I'm Catholic, I'm not active in my church. I want you to know that I've struggled for years with my decision. Eventually I met a priest who has helped me realize that I have been forgiven by God, but I still struggle with forgiving myself for my abortions.

It wasn't until I was in my thirties that I finally understood what I had actually done—I took away two lives. Sorry to sound so morbid, but that is what I felt I did. Yes, for women, I believe all options need to be fully considered and available, including the choice of abortion. If other women feel abortion is right for them, then they should have an abortion, but for me, abortion has left a lifelong emotional, spiritual, and psychological scar that I never really anticipated.

My advice to anyone who becomes pregnant when she did not intend to do so is to seek out help. Get emotional support and guidance from someone who is older, someone you trust. Get information on *all* your options. Fully embrace the decision-making process. Much later in life, self-doubts and second-guessing could arise. But if you know you undertook this decision-making process in a responsible way, then it can be the foundation that helps you avoid, or maybe simply minimize, such feelings of doubt and painful remorse. This is what I wish I had done.

RECAP

Courtney had sex without using birth control, and like so many other young women, became pregnant. Courtney also found out that the rhythm method is not a reliable way to prevent a pregnancy. Courtney was older and in college. Being older, however, does not mean that you are any more emotionally prepared to deal with the consequences of sexual intercourse. Courtney experienced the same feelings that other young women experience when they have an unintended pregnancy. Having sex for the wrong reasons can be confusing and can lead to an unintended pregnancy. Courtney thought that by having sex she and her boyfriend would get back together. They didn't, and Courtney had another unintended pregnancy. That time Steve would not help her out and she had to make the decision by herself.

Courtney gives good advice. When you are experiencing something as traumatic as an unintended pregnancy, it's best not to isolate yourself. Getting emotional support will ease some of the pain you are feeling. Deciding what to do about your pregnancy is an important decision to make. Getting all the help and support you can will make your decision process easier. It will also increase the likelihood that you will make the best decision for yourself right at this point in your life. As Courtney points out, making a sound decision now will help prevent feelings of self-doubt and second-guessing later on. Courtney wishes she had done things differently. She did not consider all her options. She has experienced feelings of remorse about her abortions for many years.

FEELINGS

Courtney felt a mix of emotions about her pregnancy. Mostly she felt alone, frightened, and overwhelmed. She was worried and scared about how her parents and her family would react to her pregnancy. She was very angry at her girlfriend for a long time for not going with her for her pregnancy test as she had promised she would do. She was in love with her boyfriend, Steve, and was hurt that he did not support her emotionally after her abortion and that he ended their relationship. She knows that she and Steve were probably not right for each other. She blamed herself for getting pregnant the second time because she did not insist that her boyfriend use birth control.

REACTIONS

Courtney's reactions were the same as many other young women who become pregnant unintentionally. She wonders what her life would have been like if she had thought through all her options and if she had placed her babies for adoption.

COPING

Being older does not mean that you will be better prepared emotionally to cope with an unintended pregnancy. An unintended pregnancy at any age can be a difficult experience. Courtney isolated herself. She didn't think she could trust anyone, so she made her decision by herself, only talking briefly about it to her boyfriend. For many years Courtney was upset about her decision. She got therapy and found a priest to whom she could talk. She still struggles with her abortions and has not fully forgiven herself.

It's important to seek help when we have pent-up, negative feelings about something we did which we feel was wrong. Discussing our feelings with someone who is objective can help. It's also important that we forgive ourselves and others for any wrong which we feel has been done. We make the best possible decisions for ourselves that we can. We can't take back what was done. All we can do is learn from it. There is no need to punish ourselves or others. Feelings of remorse, self-hate, and anguish only make us feel worse and prevent us from fully enjoying life.

9

Case Studies:
Placing a Child for Adoption

In this chapter Monica and Carolyn share their experiences. They both became pregnant at a time in their lives when they didn't want to. Monica was twenty years old at the time of her pregnancy, and Carolyn was sixteen. Monica had another daughter of whom she no longer had custody. She was also recovering from a major depression. Carolyn was in high school, and although she had the support of her parents, she did not have her boyfriend's support to raise her baby. Monica and Carolyn both chose to place their babies for adoption. They both spent a long time considering their options. The reasons they chose adoption were very similar. Both were opposed to abortion, both did not feel that at that time in their lives they were ready to be good mothers, and both wanted their children to have two parents. They both felt they made the right decision for their children and for themselves.

Monica

Monica became pregnant with her second child when she was twenty years old. She knew about birth control and she knew about parenting: Monica was nineteen when she had her first baby, Cassidy. Monica talks openly and candidly about her pregnancies, the decisions she made, and her feelings. Monica shares her story hoping that it will help someone who is in the same situation.

172

I placed my son for adoption and had a very positive experience. I am very happy with my decision. I know I made the right decision for my son. I don't have any regrets. It was a very difficult decision for me to make, but it was the right decision both for my son and for me.

I was devastated when I found out I was pregnant. I had been throwing up a lot, and feeling quite ill for a while, so I went to the emergency room. I thought I was sick with the flu, that they could give me some medication and I would get better. It was the emergency room doctor who told me I was pregnant. I was shocked. It never entered my mind that I could be pregnant. I knew the signs of pregnancy because I had been pregnant the year before. Looking back, I guess I just blocked it out. I was out of it at the time. I had just finished treatment for a major depression. I was living in a transitional home. I was just beginning to get my life together. I love children, but at that time I felt my pregnancy was ill-timed.

I was very disappointed in myself for getting pregnant. I felt stupid, like I should have known better. I was supposed to be getting my life together and instead I got pregnant. I was very angry with myself. I kept thinking, Why now? Why did I let this happen? I should have known better. I was distraught. I felt very vulnerable. My emotions were all over the place. I knew I needed support to get me through my pregnancy.

Someone from my church had told me about a special residential support program for people of all ages who are recovering from depression. For a year you live and work on a farm. Because you're secluded you can focus on yourself without the daily pressures of life. The program sounded perfect. I had known about the program for a long time, but I kept putting off looking into it. The day I found out I was pregnant I called the group. Because of my pregnancy they sped up the application process. Within one week of my call I was living at the farm.

As soon as I got there I knew I was in the right place. It was a wonderful experience to be among families, married women and men and their kids, as well as single women and single pregnant women. It wasn't an easy program because I was dealing with other issues that were not related to my pregnancy.

They had a special residence where all the single pregnant women lived. Even though we were all going through the same thing, we were not allowed to discuss our plans with each other. I absolutely did not feel any pressure from anyone about what to do or not to do.

My counselor was wonderful. She was young like me. She was like a friend. She listened to me. She was very objective. I trusted her. She wanted me to make a decision that I was comfortable with. She wanted me to think about all my options. Abortion was never an option for me. I don't believe in it, although I wouldn't discourage another woman from having one if that's what she thought was best for her. I worked through the pros and the cons of parenting versus adoption. For two months I wrote down how I felt about each option. Even though in the back of my mind I knew adoption was right for me, going through the process was very helpful. It made things concrete in my mind. It became very clear to me that adoption was the best decision I could make for my baby and myself.

There were a lot of reasons why I did not feel I could choose parenting. First of all, I was recovering from a major depression. I didn't have a job. I didn't have a place to live. Before I came to the farm I was living in transitional housing. It was temporary. They would not have allowed me to live there with a baby. The baby's father wasn't in the picture. Our relationship lasted about two months. We had broken up before I found out I was pregnant. He didn't know about my pregnancy. I wasn't in the frame of mind to be in a relationship either, so I never bothered to look him up and tell him I was pregnant. My parents would absolutely not help me with this baby. They had just taken custody of my daughter. At their age they could not take on another child. Thinking about these reasons, I knew I could not physically, emotionally, or financially be a parent.

Even if I could get all the financial resources I needed, I had serious doubts about my ability to be a good mother. I had had a taste of what parenting was all about. I didn't think I had done a good job with my daughter. Other people thought I was doing okay, but I didn't. My daughter was never neglected. She was always fed, clothed, and diapered. But she was never nurtured. Looking back on it, I knew I could have done better. I was tremendously depressed at the time. My parents knew I wanted to get control of my life, so they offered to take custody of my daughter. My parents got legal custody of Cassidy when she was one and they still have legal custody of her today.

My depression actually started when I was fifteen. I never got treatment for my depression and it got progressively worse. I was just beginning to feel better when I got pregnant again. I was at a crucial stage in my recovery. I couldn't risk failing at motherhood again. I was not going to take that chance.

The fact that my parents have legal custody of my daughter is still a difficult issue for me. It gives me a lot of comfort knowing Cassidy is loved and well cared for by my parents, but at the same time, it also hurts and causes me a great deal of pain knowing that they may never give custody back to me. I'm just beginning to realize now that there are consequences to every decision you make. At the time I made the best decision for her and for me. My only regret about that decision is that she's not with me. Right now I'm much more mature and able to be a good parent. My parents can use her as a pawn over me to get me to do what they want. Cassidy has brought a lot of love into our lives. She has changed our lives, and for the better. My parents are honest with her. They tell her that I'm her mother, and that they are her grandparents. I'm not going to be selfish. I will not disrupt Cassidy's life now even though I know I am capable of being a good mother.

So much had happened in my life by the time of my second pregnancy. My baby deserved to be loved and cared for by two people who were really ready and wanted to be parents. I owed it to myself to get better physically and emotionally. For all these reasons I chose to place my baby for adoption.

I was five months pregnant when I felt pretty comfortable with my decision to place my baby for adoption. My counselor referred me to Bethany Christian Services and I got assigned to an adoption counselor from that agency. She got together with me regularly for the next two months. She explained the adoption process, the legalities, and the emotional aspect of adoption. She was very thorough. She never pressured me. I felt that she had my best interests at heart. She wanted me to be sure that adoption was the right option for me. If I had changed my mind, she would have referred me to other community services to help me with parenting.

My adoption counselor would not let me pick the adoptive couple until she was convinced that adoption was what I wanted to do. It wasn't until I was about seven months pregnant that I reviewed profiles of potential adoptive parents. In all, I reviewed four profiles. I picked the first profile I read because they seemed like real people. They were Christians. They were in their mid-thirties. They had already adopted one son and they very much wanted another son. They owned their own business. She was a part-time school teacher.

I met the adoptive couple when I was eight-and-a-half months pregnant. Overall the meeting was intensely emotional. It was an uncomfortable experience for all of us. The adoptive mother started crying. She kept thanking me. I never cried. I feel even though the meeting was emotional it helped me. I knew as soon as I met them that they would be good parents for my baby. I didn't have questions for them. Their marriage seemed very stable. They seemed like such good people. I also trusted the agency. They had a very thorough screening process. My baby was biracial, and the parents had to go through an additional screening process before being approved. They didn't just take my son because he was next on the list. They wanted to be his parents. After the meeting, my adoption plans became more of a reality. It confirmed everything in my mind.

The adoptive parents did not come to the hospital when I gave birth. They knew that was the only time I would have with my baby. They didn't want to invade my space. I had my own room and my son stayed with me the entire time. We had four days together. Because I was placing my baby for adoption, the hospital let me stay a little longer. My hospital stay was a very positive experience. My midwife was with me and the nurses were great. Everyone kept telling me I was brave and courageous. This surprised me because that's not how I felt. I felt like I was being responsible. To give your baby a stable home with loving parents, which is something you can't give him, is responsible. I feel I did the most responsible thing I could do.

I loved my baby like he was going to go home with me. I bathed him, I fed him, and I rocked him. I even named my baby son. It made me feel good that the adoptive parents kept his first name. Sometimes I wish I had breastfed my baby. I bottlefed him because I felt that was better for him. Rejection is a big thing for me. I never wanted my child to feel rejected or abandoned. So I loved him the whole time he was inside of me. I did this by taking very good care of myself, by talking, and reading to him from the Bible. I experienced a period of peace in my second trimester which lasted the rest of my pregnancy. I decided the baby was not going to be mine, but would be someone else's. I wanted my son to be healthy. I considered this a gift to my son and to his adoptive parents. My son was healthy. He weighed seven and a half pounds and was twenty inches long.

I said my good-byes at the hospital. It was hard to say good-bye, but it wasn't that difficult. I had worked through my grief while I was pregnant. I prepared myself emotionally for the day when I would say my final good-bye. Sure, it was a loss. But the gains were far greater for me. The fact that my baby would be loved and would have two parents, a brother, and a stable home helped me a lot. I had support from my midwife and my counselors. I took a long time to make my decision and I felt comfortable with it.

The drive home and the first week home from the hospital were the hardest times. I could still feel the physical signs of birth. During that week I dreamed about the baby. My mind would wander at night. I would have those annoying "what if" questions, like, "What if the couple conned everyone? What if they really weren't a loving couple?" I talked all these feelings over with my counselor. She explained to me that they were all normal. Even though I had these dreams, I never regretted my decision. I have always felt that I made the best decision for myself and my baby.

My baby lived with another family for the first three weeks of his life. This is called "neutral care." It mainly protected me in case I wanted to change my mind. It also protected the adoptive parents in case they changed their minds. I never changed my mind. There were times I wished the baby was with me. That was the mothering instinct in me. Whenever this happened, I would remind myself that I made the best decision for my baby and myself. I didn't have what it took to be a good mother, what my baby needed and deserved.

After three weeks went by, I signed the final adoption papers. It was a very closed, private meeting among the court-appointed lawyer, the judge, and myself. My counselors came with me too. It wasn't a bad experience. I remember thinking, This is all so permanent. But then I would remind myself that this was a part of adoption, which I accepted. The support from my two counselors really helped me.

The adoptive parents sent me pictures and another letter when my son was six months old, and a letter when he was one year old. After the second letter I asked them not to contact me anymore. I was trying to get on with my life. I explained to them that my son was always in my thoughts and prayers, but getting the updates was too painful for me. I had made my decision. I felt comfortable with my decision. The updates were upsetting me. It was like I had a scar which kept reopening. I kept reliving the loss. They will only send updates to the adoption file. That way they will stay on record for me at the adoption agency. I can read them if I change my mind.

By state law my son can look me up when he turns twenty-one. The adoptive parents told me they will be very honest with him about his adoption and about me. I wrote my son a letter. I told him about my decision and that I loved him. I never told him anything but the truth. The letter will stay in his file at the adoption agency. He can read it when he turns twenty-one. I hope that when he turns twenty-one he will look me up, but I won't push for a meeting. If he doesn't want to look me up I'll have to deal with it then. I'm not going to worry now about something that may or may not happen for so long.

I know there are people who may not agree with what I did. Some people would not agree no matter what I did. I do not share my adoption with everyone. People may reject me because of what I did—I knew that when I made my decision. That didn't change my mind. People can reject you for any reason, whether they think you should have had an abortion or parented your child. That's just part of life. I was thinking about my baby. Planning what was best for my baby became more important to me than what other people thought. Sure, my child may reject me when he turns twenty-one. I will have to deal with it then. I can die right now and know I made the right decision.

Overall my experience was very positive. I have no regrets about my decision. Because my experience was so positive, I don't want anyone to think that it was something that could only happen on TV. My decision was hard to make. My feelings and emotions were very intense. I knew it would be very hard, but it was not impossible. I got through it with lots of help and support from people who loved and cared about me.

I did most of my grieving while I was pregnant. I worked out all my feelings with both my adoption counselor and my counselor at the farm. My adoption counselor stayed in touch with me for two years. She wanted to make sure I was doing okay. I liked that. I was feeling some pain with my loss, but it got better. I feel the pain goes away and that you can get on with your life as long as you're willing to work through your feelings.

What helped me was knowing that I made the decision and that it was the best decision for my baby and myself. No one else made the decision for me. No one pressured me. When I first chose adoption, I thought I would have no control, that the agency would select my baby's parents. It was just the opposite. I picked the parents. I had control over the adoption process.

My advice to other young women is to work with an agency that cares about you. Work through your feelings with someone who specializes in loss and grieving. See your counselor before and after your delivery. As an outsider your counselor can be objective and can help you progress through the various stages of grieving. If you are feeling some pain, whether or not you have a history of depression, it will only get worse if you don't deal with it.

I left the farm after a year feeling like a new person. I was emotionally and physically stronger. I moved to another area. Two years later I met a man whom I love very much. He wanted very much to have a child. I felt in a better position to have a baby. I'm twenty-four now, and I just had my second baby girl. In a few months I am going to complete my cosmetology license. I had started it when I was in high school, but never finished it. This time I am going to finish it so I have something for myself and a way to support our daughter.

RECAP

Monica chose adoption because she felt it was the best decision for her baby and herself. She was opposed to abortion, so her options were to raise her baby or place him for adoption. She carefully weighed the pros and cons of each. Monica had a daughter when she was nineteen. She was now twenty and her parents had just received custody of her daughter. This caused Monica some pain. Monica was recovering from a major depression. At that time, even though she had already graduated from high school, she felt she wasn't able to raise her baby. She did not feel she could physically, emotionally, or financially support her baby. Monica wanted her baby to have a stable home with two parents. She knew she couldn't provide that for her baby, so she chose adoption. Monica actively participated in the adoption process; she even chose the adoptive parents.

FEELINGS

Monica was devastated when she found out she was pregnant. Even though she had been pregnant before she didn't recognize her pregnancy symptoms. Monica was recovering from a major depression. She didn't have emotional support from the baby's father. Her parents were willing to provide her emotional support no matter what she chose to do. However, they would not help her financially or help her care for her baby. She felt vulnerable and alone.

Monica worked through much of her grief while she was pregnant. She experienced a sense of peace after she made her decision to place her baby for adoption. Monica enjoyed the second and third trimester of her pregnancy. She enjoyed the changes in her body. She took very good care of herself physically and spiritually while she was pregnant. She felt very connected to the baby growing in her womb.

Monica felt pain when the family continued to contact her during the baby's first year of life, but she does not regret her decision. She feels she did what was best for her baby and herself.

REACTIONS

Monica acted quickly when she discovered she was pregnant. She knew she needed help to make her decision. She knew she did not want to be alone during her pregnancy. Monica knew about a supportive residence which she called the day she found out she was pregnant. Monica moved there within a week. She relied on her counselors for emotional support with her decision.

COPING

Monica knew she had other issues which she needed to resolve in her life when she became pregnant. She relied on counselors to help her not only with her depression, but also through the decision-making process. She also relied on the support of other people with whom she was living, who were also dealing with depression and other crises in their lives. Monica controlled the adoption process. She picked out the parents. She wrote a letter to her baby. She ended contact with the adoptive parents when she realized it was too painful for her.

Monica enjoyed her pregnancy. She worked through much of her grief while she was pregnant. She took very good care of herself during her pregnancy because this was one of the best things she could do for her baby. She took pride in the fact that she was giving her baby the gift of good health, as well as giving the adoptive parents the gift of a healthy baby. Monica still thinks about her baby. She wonders what he looks like. But she finds comfort knowing that he lives in a good home with loving parents and a brother.

Three years after the adoption, Monica had a baby girl with someone she loves. She now feels she is a good mother, and that she is emotionally able to be a good parent. She is working on her cosmetology license so she can help support her baby.

Carolyn

> Carolyn became pregnant when she was sixteen. She knew all about birth control. She had been taking the pill for a year.

I was finishing my sophomore year in high school when I found out I was pregnant. My boyfriend was graduating from high school. I kept forgetting to take my pills. I knew I was supposed to use back-up protection, but I didn't bother. I was preoccupied with our relationship. My boyfriend, Dave, had just received a football scholarship from a college on the West Coast. I knew it would be hard for us to get together and I was worried that our relationship wouldn't last.

When I missed my period, I went right away to a clinic with my best friend. I knew I was pregnant all along, but was afraid to find out. I cried and cried when the nurse told me I was pregnant. I couldn't believe that I had let this happen. I had been on the pill for about a year, and until I was preoccupied about Dave leaving, I was always responsible about taking it. I felt good about that. But when I found out I was pregnant, I was devastated. I thought I had been so stupid to have forgotten to take my pills. I could have prevented the pregnancy. I blamed myself. I should have known better. My first reaction was that I would raise my baby. Some of my friends have had abortions, and I didn't want to have one. I don't think it's right.

I told my boyfriend right away that I was pregnant. I was totally unprepared for his response. We had dated for over a year. He wanted me to go to the same college so we could be together. Dave said he wasn't ready to be a parent; he couldn't handle the responsibility. He had assumed we would travel together after college. He didn't want to have kids for a while. He reminded me of my goals and told me I should continue my education without being burdened with a child. He wanted me to have an abortion and offered to pay for it. I was very upset with him. I couldn't believe that he assumed I would have an abortion. He wouldn't talk to me after I told him I was planning on raising our child. He was very clear that he would not support me financially or emotionally.

I was an emotional wreck after our talk. I cried for a few days. I finally got the courage to talk to my parents. They knew something was wrong because I hadn't been myself for a while. My parents were shocked. My mother cried. My dad got very angry. He threatened to call Dave's parents. My parents were so upset that we all agreed to talk the next night.

My parents were great once they got over their initial shock. They talked to me about all my options. They told me they would support me no matter what choice I made. They reminded me that I was an honor student and that I had always wanted to go to college and be an international journalist. They understood why I didn't want to have an abortion. They were willing to help if I decided to parent my child. They told me they would pay for the baby's medical care and day care so I could continue with school. They were clear about what they were not willing to do. They would not babysit. They told me I would have to get a part-time job to pay for clothes, diapers, and a babysitter for when I wanted to go out with my friends.

I thought about all my options over and over. I knew it would be difficult to raise a child even with my parents' help. I wanted to go to college and have a career. I had always dreamed of living in a foreign country before settling down and having children. I began to think more and more about adoption. My cousin was adopted. We are the same age. She has a good relationship with her parents, my aunt and uncle. She told me she wonders why her birth mother placed her for adoption, but she doesn't spend a lot of time thinking about it. She just figures her birth mother couldn't raise her by herself and wanted her to have two parents.

I asked my parents to bring me to a local adoption agency. My adoption counselor was very helpful. She told me she wanted me to make a decision which was right for me. She never pressured me to choose adoption. She arranged for me to speak to another teen who placed her baby for adoption. I felt better after hearing about her experience.

I made the mistake of telling my best friend about my plans. She freaked out. She started yelling at me, accusing me of being irresponsible. She told me I would always regret my decision. She's my best friend. I was really hurt by what she said. I thought she was open-minded and had liberal views. Wow, was I shocked! I never anticipated how she would react. I was counting on her to be more supportive of me. I thought about what she said. I could have raised my child with my parents' support, but that wasn't what I wanted to do. I felt it wasn't fair for my child to grow up without a father. I wanted my child to have a better life than what I was able to give. I knew it would be hard for me to get my education. I wasn't emotionally ready to be a parent. The more I thought about it, adoption made the most sense.

I picked out the adoptive couple. I looked at profiles of lots of adoptive couples. The couple I chose were in their late thirties. They had both gone to college. They were smart. They had good jobs and both spoke another language. They were athletic and had a pet dog. They were the kind of parents I would want to be for my child. They had been trying for years to have a child. I could have met them in person, but I didn't want to. I thought the meeting would be too painful for me.

The summer was almost over. I was beginning to look pregnant. I told my parents I couldn't go back to the same school. I couldn't handle being judged by my classmates. My parents made arrangements for me to live with an aunt in another state. I could have gone to a special school for pregnant teens, but I decided against it. I wasn't willing to take the risk of having my friends find out about my pregnancy. I was fearful they would reject me. I had a home tutor until after I delivered the baby. My counselor helped me find a support group of other teens who were placing their babies for adoption. I think that helped prepare me for my delivery.

My mom and dad came for the delivery. My mom was my labor coach. I had a baby girl. I fed and bathed my baby, and named her Susan, after my grandmother. The nurses told me my baby was beautiful. They let me spend as much time as I wanted with Susan.

Dave never came to the hospital. I wasn't surprised, because there had been a lot of tension between us. I was angry and hurt by him because he wasn't interested in raising our baby.

I left my baby at the hospital. That was very difficult for me to do. I felt very sad and empty inside. I signed the adoption papers as soon as I legally could. I wanted Susan to be with her adoptive family as soon as possible. I didn't want to have any delays.

I stayed at my aunt's house for the rest of the school year. I took night classes. I even took extra language classes. I got a part-time job and saved my money. I stayed very busy. I blocked the whole experience out of my mind. With the money I earned from my job and also with the help of my parents, I was able to travel to Mexico with a youth group for a month in the summer.

After the trip, I went back to live with my parents. In the fall I returned to my old high school. It was my senior year. I didn't tell anyone about my baby. My best friend didn't tell anyone, even though she disagreed with what I did. I made up a story that I spent a year as an exchange student in Mexico. I kept very busy. I applied to several colleges, and got accepted to my first choice.

I started feeling funny around the time of my baby's first birthday. I was crying a lot. My parents brought me to see the counselor from the adoption agency. She told me my feelings were normal. She explained to me that it is typical to have a reaction around the baby's birthday and to feel sad when I think of her. Knowing that my feelings were normal helped me to feel better. She helped me see that I hadn't grieved the loss of my baby, that I had just blocked it out. My counselor helped me realize that I was still angry at my boyfriend for leaving me and at myself for getting pregnant. She helped me see that my anger was preventing me from feeling good about my decision. She helped me make a plan. I wrote a letter to myself. I wrote down all my feelings. It took me hours. I wrote about how I felt the first time Dave kissed me. I wrote about how I felt when he bailed out on me. Then I wrote about the adoption. When I finished I went to a river behind my house. I made sailboats out of each page of my letter. I put them in the water and watched them drift off. I cried the whole time. I was exhausted by the time I was done. But I felt tremendous relief.

It's been three years since the birth of my baby. I'm now a sophomore in college. I still feel sad around my baby's birthday, but the pain is much more manageable. Now when I feel sad, I do something good for myself. I remind myself that I made the best choice for myself and my baby. I feel good about myself, that I was able to make a plan and carry through with it. I find comfort knowing that my baby is being raised by a loving couple. I believe I made the right decision for myself and for my baby. If I had to do it again, I would still choose adoption. I want to have a child someday, but not until I've finished school and I'm married. I plan to place my name with a birth registry. That way Susan can look me up when she turns eighteen if she wants to. She will know where I am. I won't look her up. I won't interfere with her life.

I just started dating one guy. We were friends for a year before we started seeing each other. I haven't told him yet about the baby. I just told him I didn't want to be pressured into having sex. He was real cool about it. We both agreed not to have sex until we are ready and know that we can handle the consequences.

RECAP

Carolyn chose adoption even though her boyfriend wanted her to have an abortion and her best friend thought she should raise her child. Carolyn thought about raising her child. Her parents offered some support, but reminded her that she was the mother and the responsible person for her child. Carolyn valued the opinion of her best friend, but she didn't change her mind even when the friend pressured her. Carolyn felt adoption was the best choice for her. She wanted her baby to have a better life than what she could provide. Carolyn actively participated in the adoption process.

FEELINGS

Carolyn was initially afraid to tell her parents. She felt better after telling them and was relieved that they did not make the decision for her. She was very hurt and angry at her boyfriend because he didn't want to raise their child together. She was angry and disappointed in her best friend because she wasn't supportive of her feelings. Carolyn held positive views about adoption and felt adoption was best for her and her baby.

Carolyn hadn't anticipated that the feelings of loss and sadness would continue even after the adoption process was complete. Many teens share this misconception. Adoption is a loss, and like all losses needs to be grieved. The grieving process is different for everyone. Most teens feel sad around their baby's birthday. This is normal.

REACTIONS

Carolyn hid her pregnancy from her friends and classmates. She lived away from home so she could keep her pregnancy a secret. She relied on her parents and her counselor for emotional support with her decision. She tried to block her feelings of loss and sadness, but it didn't work and she ended up being depressed.

COPING

Carolyn coped with her feelings of loss and sadness through the help of her counselor. Her counselor helped her realize that her feelings were normal and that acknowledging her emotions was a healthy way to cope with her loss. Her counselor helped her deal positively with her anger. As Carolyn began dealing with her anger, she felt less depressed. Through the help of her counselor she found a support group of other teens who were in the same situation.

Carolyn still thinks about her baby and is still sad that she is not raising Susan, but she feels better because she knows that she made the best decision for herself and for her baby. She wants to have another child someday, but she plans on waiting until she's emotionally and financially ready to be a parent.

10

Your Partner's Responsibility

. . . Ain't no doubt about it, we were doubly blessed. We were barely seventeen and we were barely dressed. . . . I've gotta let you know, no you're never gonna regret it, so open up your heart. I've got a big surprise. It'll be all right. . . .

Stop right there, I've gotta know right now, before we go any further. Do you love me? Will you love me forever? Do you need me? Will you never leave me? Will you make me so happy for the rest of my life? Will you take me away? Will you make me your wife? Do you love me? Will you love me forever? Do you need me? Will you never leave me? . . . I've gotta know right now, before we go any further. Do you love me? Will you love me forever?

Let me sleep on it. Baby, Baby, let me sleep on it. . . . I'll give you an answer in the morning. . . .

—*Meat Loaf, "Paradise by the Dashboard Light"*

Sara was crying. She and Andy had been talking about what she should do and it had been an emotional conversation. Sara hadn't made her final decision yet. She had hoped that Andy would have had a change of heart, that once they got together again, Andy would change his mind. She had asked Andy to move back home and go to a local college; that way he could help her out with the baby. She told Andy that she wanted her baby to have a father. She wanted his emotional support. She didn't expect him to help her out financially until after he graduated from college. Andy felt bad and said, "Sara, we made a mistake. We got carried away. I'm sorry Sara. I'm just not ready to be a father now. I want to date other people. You should too. How will you finish high school? How will you go to college? Don't you think you're being unfair to your mom, with everything she's going through?" Andy wanted Sara to consider adoption. Sara was hurt and angry with Andy. Their relationship was not going to continue; Sara knew she was on her own. The decision was hers to make. If she decided to raise their baby, she knew that she would be doing it on her own. Andy would only support her financially, and that wasn't what she wanted. The idea of being a single mother frightened her.

More teenagers are sexually active today than in previous years. When you're sexually active there's *always* the risk of a pregnancy, because *contraceptive measures are not 100 percent effective*. Some teens, like Sara and Andy, make the mistake of not using any birth control. If you do not use birth control, you are at a high risk of getting pregnant. Sara got pregnant the first time she had sex, which was also Andy's first sexual experience. A pregnancy was something that Sara and Andy did not anticipate. Studies have shown that the vast majority of pregnant teens and their partners did not plan their pregnancy.

Sara and Andy have a big decision to make. Today teen pregnancies are handled much differently than they were in the past. Years ago, when a young woman became pregnant she would often marry. Back then, a young man knew it was expected of him to marry the young woman whose child he fathered. If he did not marry her the young woman secretly had an abortion or placed her baby for adoption. Single parenthood was not socially acceptable, and as a result was not as common then as it is today. Although marriage is one option, fewer teens today are getting married. A young man is reluctant to marry today because he doesn't have an established career or a way to support himself and his family. Recent statistics indicate that only three out of ten teen moms marry.[1] Marriage isn't your only option, and it may not be your best option. Teen marriages tend to be very unstable, and have a high divorce rate. Fortunately today there are other options available to you and your boyfriend.

Single parenting is more socially acceptable today. You and your boyfriend can raise your child together without getting married. However, you and your boyfriend may also decide you don't want to raise your child. You don't have to raise your child now if that's something you both don't feel you can do. You and your boyfriend can continue your relationship and place your baby for adoption or terminate the pregnancy. You may also agree to end your relationship, like Sara and Andy did. If this happens, you will be left to make a decision in the same way that Sara was.

Andy and Sara reached an agreement, although neither one was completely happy about it. Andy would prefer that Sara place their baby for adoption, but he agreed to help out financially in some way if Sara chose to raise their baby. Sara would continue her pregnancy, but she hadn't decided whether she would raise their baby or place it for adoption.

As Sara and Andy found out, when an unintended pregnancy happens there can be conflict and a lot of hurt feelings. Like Sara you must make a decision which will have a big impact on your life, your boyfriend's life, and your families' lives. Conflict can arise because you and your boyfriend may not agree on how to resolve your pregnancy. You or your boyfriend may want more of a commitment than the other person is willing to give. If expectations are not met, someone may end up feeling hurt. Sara was concerned about raising her child alone. She didn't want to do that. She wanted to continue their relationship and wanted Andy to take an active role in parenting their child. She had expectations of Andy which he was not willing to fulfill. Andy agreed to provide some financial support; however, Andy didn't want the responsibility of parenting their child. He didn't want to continue their relationship. As a result, Sara felt hurt, alone, and confused about what she should do.

It's hard to say how your boyfriend will react to your pregnancy. How he reacts may have a lot to do with how long you've been in a relationship, what his personal plans are for his life right now, and how he feels parenting now will affect those plans. Research has shown that most adult men want to become a father at some point in their life. However, the majority of young men do not want to begin fatherhood during their teen years. One recent study which asked young men how they would feel about becoming a father during their teen years revealed some interesting findings: only 4 percent of young men reported that they would be "very pleased" about becoming a father, whereas 69 percent said they would be "very upset."[2]

The vast majority of these young men said that they should worry about impregnating a young woman even though she could terminate her pregnancy. The majority of the young men indicated that they would behave responsibly if their girlfriend became pregnant. Here's what they said:

- 88 percent of the young men agreed that a young man is equally responsible for his child
- 95 percent agreed that they would have to give the mother money for the baby

Here's what Ryan had to say when he found out his girlfriend, Danielle, was pregnant:

> Danielle and I had been seeing each other for a couple of years when she got pregnant. Danielle really wanted to have the baby but I wasn't so sure about being a father yet. It was something I assumed we'd always do, but not this soon. I was eager to do the right thing, so I went along with Danielle. I'm being responsible. It's not easy for me. I'm going to school and juggling a part-time job. I give her some money to support our baby. It's not a lot, but it's the best I can do right now. I also help out taking care of our son.

Another young man was quite eager to be a father. He reacted with enthusiasm when his girlfriend told him she suspected she was pregnant. However, his girlfriend had no intentions of being a mother at that time in her life. Here's what Stacey, a college freshman, had to say about what happened to her:

> I'll never forget the expression on my boyfriend's face when I told him I thought I was pregnant. He had a grin from ear to ear. He was so happy. He got down on his hands and knees and proposed. I panicked. I told him, "No way, you got it all wrong. This is a mistake. I'm not ready to be a mother." My parents had gone through a messy divorce the year before, and then my dad died suddenly. Marriage was like a terminal disease to me. I couldn't understand why anyone would get married. I loved Chris. But we had only known each other for about six months. I didn't feel like I was emotionally ready to be a good mother yet. I wanted a career and to travel before I settled down. Lucky for me it was a pregnancy scare. It changed my life. I've always been very responsible and careful about contraception from that point on.

All young men do not react to their girlfriend's pregnancies with the same enthusiasm. Some young men are angry when their girlfriend becomes pregnant. They struggle with their feelings. Sometimes young men buy into the idea that sexual freedom is part of growing up. They have a lot of anger and confusion when they have to be responsible about a pregnancy that they didn't intend to happen. Here's what Richard had to say when he found out that his girlfriend, Renee, was pregnant:

> I was just having a good time. Isn't that what everyone my age is doing? Sure, I like my girlfriend, but there's no future in our relationship. No way am I ready to settle down yet. We had only been going together for about

a month when she got pregnant. She wants me to do something. I'm mad. She knows we were just having a good time. Everyone tells you to have fun when you're young. No one tells you ahead of time about responsibility. It's not fair. Being a father, commitment, and marriage are the last things on my mind.

Sometimes a young man questions whether he's the father of his baby. There are some young men who mistakenly believe that they could never get a girl pregnant, even if they had not used birth control. They react with shock and anger to the news of a pregnancy. Sometimes they even deny that they are the father. Here's what James had to say:

A girl I had been going with told me I was the father of her child. I went off on her. Why should I believe her? How am I supposed to know for sure that I'm the father of her baby? I'm dating other people. She's been dating other people. I told her to find the real father.

You may be angry with your boyfriend if he does not respond to your pregnancy the way you would like him to. His response may not make sense to you. Unfortunately, young men and young women often approach sex differently. Their opinions about sex and their interest in it can be quite different. Young men are more likely than young women to say that they think and talk about sex more often. Boys tend to begin having sex at an earlier age than girls. Also, historically, there's a big difference in the way young men and young women are socialized to think and behave about sex. Oftentimes a young man is encouraged by his older brother, father, or male friends to go out and "sow his wild oats," or to "score" as much as he wants. Not all young men buy into this. However, some do. They view sex at this time in their life as a way of having a "good time." If their girlfriend becomes pregnant, they may react with anger and confusion, like Richard did. They may struggle with whether or not they want the responsibility of fatherhood at this time in their life.

Sometimes sex has a very different meaning for a young woman than it does for a young man. Young women are socialized to feel very differently about sex. For starters, they worry that their reputation will be ruined if word gets around that they've been sexually active. Young women have to deal with the consequences of a pregnancy, and tend to worry more about the possibility of getting pregnant. In addition, young women tend to view sex as a way of experiencing emotional closeness as well as establishing and maintaining a relationship with a young man. In other words, many women focus mainly on the emotional side of sex, and many men focus mainly on the physical aspects.

Perhaps you have the same views as the woman in the song by Meat Loaf does. This woman wants a guarantee of a commitment before she has sex with her boyfriend. Some young women assume that if they have sex with their boyfriend then that means they're in a committed relationship. That may not be the case. Your boyfriend may have entirely different views about sex, relationships, and responsibility. If you had sex with your boyfriend because you were looking for emotional closeness or a commitment from him and you're not getting that, you may feel hurt and used. If you're like Sara and your boyfriend doesn't want to be a father, you may feel devastated. Your pregnancy does not mean that you and your boyfriend will automatically stay together.

Courtney thought she would get back together with her ex-boyfriend by having sex with him. Recall what Courtney had to say:

> Steve told me that he held me fully responsible for the pregnancy this second time, and would not "support" me in any way. We clearly were not boyfriend/girlfriend then. This sexual encounter was a one-night stand kind of thing. . . . I also felt responsible for the pregnancy . . . I actually used sex to re-engage him in a relationship. I acted irresponsibly by not using birth control. I got pregnant and we never got back together again. . . .

It's best to be open and honest with your boyfriend when you discuss your pregnancy. You will want to know exactly what you can expect of your boyfriend should you choose to raise your child. If your boyfriend's opinion will influence your decision, then there's an even more important reason to be honest with him. According to the Alan Guttmacher Institute, over three-fourths of pregnant teens talk over their decision with their boyfriend.

Involving your boyfriend with your decision-making process benefits him. Teen dads frequently have difficulty coping with the news of their girlfriend's pregnancy. They must consider the same things that you need to consider. Your pregnancy is bound to stir up a mix of emotions in your boyfriend. He will experience a lot of stress worrying about how the pregnancy will affect his life, his relationship with you, and whether or not he's emotionally and financially ready to be a parent. One study found that teen dads who were included in their partner's decision-making process experienced fewer symptoms of anxiety or depression. Teen dads who suffered the most were those who did not want the pregnancy, who were not included in the decision-making process, and were not sure about what to do. Here's what Mark had to say when he found out his girlfriend, Julie, was pregnant:

> At first I was happy and excited when I found out I was going to be a father. I was seventeen and a junior in high school. I was never a good student. I was already behind one year in school. I was finally feeling like I was catching up when my girlfriend got pregnant. I had mixed emotions. I was angry at myself because I hadn't used birth control and was also angry at my girlfriend for getting pregnant. I felt confused about what to do. I thought my social life was over. I worried about how I was going to be able to support a baby. My girlfriend and I went to our mothers for advice. My mom was real mad at me. She felt I was too young to be a father. My girlfriend's mother offered to help us out. My girlfriend and I made the decision to be parents together. It's a decision I feel good about. I know my girlfriend will make a terrific mom, and with her mother's help we'll be okay. We're both in this together.

Ron's girlfriend, Jocelyn, told him about her pregnancy, but ultimately made a decision with which he did not agree. Ron suffered a lot by this, and was very distressed by what his girlfriend had done. This is what Ron had to say:

> My girlfriend told me she was pregnant as soon as she found out. At first I was shocked. I distanced myself from her for a while. I was having a hard time trying to decide what to do. I'm Catholic and don't believe in abortion, but at the same time it didn't seem to make sense for us to be parents. I certainly didn't feel ready to be a father. It took me a couple of weeks to get a hold of my feelings. During that time I got a lot of advice from different people. After a while, I started getting used to the idea of being a father. When I went to talk to her, she had already made up her mind to have an abortion. She wouldn't change her mind even after I told her how I felt. She said if I had really wanted to be a father, I would have known right away. She couldn't handle my initial uncertainty. She had an abortion within a week of our conversation. I was really hurt by what she did. She told me if I really cared about her I'd agree with her decision. I think we would have made good parents. I didn't feel right about our relationship or about her after that. I couldn't deal with what she did. I ended our relationship.

Some young women do not tell their partners about their pregnancy and make the decision completely on their own. Sometimes a young woman realizes she's pregnant after a relationship has ended, and other times she has her own reasons for not wanting to involve her boyfriend. It's up to you whether or not you involve your boyfriend with your decision-making process. If you make your decision on your own, you will have to deal with the consequences of how he will feel and react if he finds out. Kate, who shares her experience in chapter 7, did not inform her boyfriend that she was pregnant. She made her decision on her own to raise their baby. Recall what Kate had to say:

> Dave was shocked when I called him to tell him about Jessica. . . . He yelled at me. He was furious at me for not telling him that I had gone off the pill. He said I had deceived him and I deserved whatever happened to me. He told me I had no right to look for support from him, since he felt I would never have gotten pregnant in the first place if I had been honest with him about being off the pill. He absolutely refused to see Jessica. . . . Dave's reaction left me feeling sad, rejected, unloved, and totally alone.

You and your boyfriend may want to take some time to decide what to do. Your boyfriend may need some time to adjust to the pregnancy and work through his feelings. This is a serious decision to make. It's wise for both of you to seek guidance and counseling from your families, a member of a religious group, a trusted adult, or a pregnancy counselor.

Deciding to be a parent is a big decision for both you and your boyfriend to make. It's not a decision to be made quickly. It requires a lot of thought. You must consider how your lives will be changed, and whether you both feel you are capable of being parents at this time in your life. If you and your boyfriend decide to raise your child together, the effect on his life will be almost as great as the effect on your own life. If you decide to be parents, it's best if you are both up front and direct with your families right away. You and your boyfriend will need their help and support. If both sets of parents won't agree to help, you may both want to reconsider your decision or find alternative resources.

There isn't a lot known about the effects of early fatherhood on teen dads. This is because to date there hasn't been a lot of research on teen dads. The male role in teenage pregnancy for years has been overlooked and has only recently begun to receive attention. One reason for this is that historically, pregnancy prevention, childbearing, and child rearing have been considered women's issues. It is the woman who becomes pregnant and who must deal with the pregnancy. Also, adolescent fathers, because they were unmarried, tended to be excluded from participating in the birth and care of their child. As a result, research on childbirth and child rearing has tended to focus almost exclusively on women.

Times are changing. In recent years, men of all ages have been encouraged to take part in their partner's labor and delivery. More fathers now participate in childbirth classes, are present at the delivery, and are taking a more active role in child rearing. At the same time, there is also growing societal concern about the effect of absent fathers on the well-being of their children. More children are living in poverty today, in large part because they are being raised in households headed by single females. At one time, an unmarried father could walk away from his responsibility to care for his child born outside of marriage. Today that is no longer possible. Changes in laws and societal opinions make it more difficult for men of all ages to do this. With this increase in public awareness of the male role in family formation and support, researchers have begun to look more closely at the role of the teen dad and the effect of early fatherhood on his life, the teen mom's life, and their baby.

One thing that is becoming apparent is that there are fewer teen dads than teen moms, although the actual number of teen dads is difficult to determine. One of the reasons for this is that young women usually date men who are two to three years older than they are. Another reason is that many teen mothers do not include the father's age on the baby's birth registration form. One study found that in 1990, only 58 percent of teen mothers revealed the age of their baby's father on the birth certificate. For the births to teen mothers where the father's age was reported, slightly less than one-third of the fathers were also under age twenty a little more than one-half were aged twenty to twenty-four.

Becoming a father at a young age can have the same negative consequences for young men as it does for young women. Early parenthood for teen dads interferes with their ability to complete their education and establish satisfactory careers. Because teen dads do not usually assume primary responsibility for their children, it's generally thought that teenage parenthood is less disruptive on young men's lives than is on young women's. Teen dads who marry and have children while still teenagers tend to be at the highest risk of experiencing difficulties. For instance, one study revealed that teen dads whose children are conceived inside of marriage drop out of school at a higher rate than either teen dads whose children are conceived out of wedlock or teen males who don't father children.[3]

Available research shows that teen dads obtain less formal education than their peers who delay parenting. Teen dads are less likely to receive a regular high school diploma, more likely to receive a General Equivalency Diploma (GED), and more likely to complete their high school education at an older age. Because teen dads enter the labor force sooner and with less education, they have difficulty finding a satisfying, well-paying job.

Many young men suffer depression and anxiety over the changes in their lives brought on by early parenting. Studies have shown that teen dads and teen moms share similarities. Teen dads also tend to be poor and have less education. A baby places an additional hardship on a teen dad and makes it even more difficult for him to get ahead. In addition, he will experience a loss in his personal freedom. His relationships with his peers will drastically change. He will not have the free time he once had to hang out with his friends. He may experience difficulty completing his education and may worry about how he will financially support his girlfriend and his child.

Besides the financial strain, a teen dad will experience stress from changes in his relationships with his family and his girlfriend's family. A young man who fathers a child is often unfairly stereotyped as exploitative, uncaring, and irresponsible. In general he is thought of as a lousy guy. He's in a situation where he very likely cannot win with his own family or with his girlfriend's family. He faces negative reactions from both sets of parents. His own and his girlfriend's families may be angry and disappointed in him. As a result, he may be rejected by both families. His girlfriend's family may not allow him to have any contact with her. If this happens, he will probably feel alone and isolated.

A teen dad will likely also be concerned about the health of his girlfriend and his baby. He may not understand the physical and psychological changes associated with pregnancy or how to care for a baby. He may sincerely want to help out and be supportive, but may not know how. Because he doesn't know much about child rearing, he may have unrealistic expectations of his baby's growth and development. He may become impatient with his child. Parenting can be stressful for him.

Even though teen dads are less likely to marry the mothers of their babies than are older men, many teen dads have regular contact with their children, at least initially, and provide some type of assistance. After the birth of their child, many young fathers have regular contact by providing direct child care and some type of financial support even though it was not court ordered.[4] However, the frequency of their contact tends to lessen over time. One study which looked at the involvement of young fathers over a twelve-year period found that about a third of the children studied had regular contact with their fathers: 17 percent lived with their dad; 16 percent lived apart but maintained regular weekly visits.[5]

You will need more than child-care assistance and emotional support from your boyfriend. You will also need financial assistance. Financial assistance is important because raising a child costs a lot of money. Your boyfriend may not be able to contribute as much as you would like. One study found that teen dads contributed to the care of their child by providing food, diapers, clothing, and some child care, as well as financial assistance. However, six out of ten of the teen mothers considered the father's contributions to his child's upbringing as not enough.[6] This is something you may also want to anticipate. Teen dads are more likely to come from financially disadvantaged backgrounds. Your boyfriend may already be experiencing difficulty supporting himself. A child will place an additional financial burden on him. If he does have a job, it's likely that it doesn't pay much because he's young and has less education. Realistically he may not be able to provide much financial support.

To get by, many single mothers rely on child support payments from the fathers of their babies. However, very few teen mothers receive such payments. A research study from 1984 found that a mother who had her first child as a teenager and who was no longer living with the baby's father had only a three in ten chance of receiving a child support payment. For mothers who were older when their first child was born, the chance was slightly better: four in ten.[7] The child support payment you receive is not likely to be very high. The Alan Guttmacher Institute reports that in 1987 the average annual child support payment for mothers under the age of thirty was only $1,946.[8] That amounts to roughly $162 a month. This really isn't a lot of money, yet it was about 22 percent of the fathers' income. The amount you receive, if any, is not likely to provide enough financial support for you. Day care alone can be a big expense. Some teens are able to get day care through their schools and some aren't. Even if you can get free or subsidized day care for your baby, it's still not cheap to raise a baby. Find out how much your boyfriend is able to contribute and see if this will be enough to support you and your baby. If it's not enough, you may also have to get a job, get help from your family, and/or apply for public assistance.

Research has shown that some young women are strongly influenced by the views of their partner. They make a decision about their pregnancy based on what their boyfriend wants them to do. If you decide to raise your baby because your partner wants you to, you may have a tough time coping if your boyfriend is not as available to you and your baby as you would like him to be. All teens mature at different ages, but in general males take longer to mature. Your boyfriend may be sincere when he tells you that he wants to be a father. He may start off with very good intentions; however, he may find that parenting is more than he can handle. He may lack the maturity and the knowledge needed to take on parenting at this time in his life. Your boyfriend may become frustrated, and as the statistics indicate, become less involved with you and your child's care. Raising a child is always a challenge. Raising a child alone when you thought you would have your boyfriend's help may be frustrating and stressful for you. You will most likely experience emotional and financial difficulties.

Raising your child without your boyfriend's support is something which you may not think will happen to you, especially if you and your boyfriend have been in a long-term relationship. You may be excited about the idea of raising your child together. It's important to keep in mind that as the mother of your child you are ultimately responsible for him or her. The burden of raising your child will always rest on your shoulders. This is true no matter how many people promise you ahead of time that they will help you out. The reality is that your boyfriend may not carry through with what he promises. There are no guarantees with any relationship that it will last. Raising your child alone, whether you marry your boyfriend or remain single, is a possibility which you should always consider. This happened to Shauna. She never anticipated raising her child on her own. It came as a big surprise to her when her boyfriend, Aaron, stopped being as involved in the care of their child. Shauna explains:

I never thought it would happen to me. My boyfriend and I had been going together for a while before I got pregnant. Aaron was thrilled when I told him I was pregnant. He begged me to have our baby. He had dropped out of school the year before, and was going to night school for his GED. He had a day-time job. He lives with his mom and two younger brothers. He adores his brothers. He's so good with them. I thought he'd make a great dad. He was there for me the whole time I was pregnant. At first he was always there for me and our daughter. When she was just a little baby he was so good with her. He was gentle and loving. As she got older and needed more attention he started getting frustrated taking care of her. He used to babysit three to four hours a week for me so I could get out. He stopped doing that a long time ago. He doesn't go to doctor's appointments with me anymore either. He helps out a little financially, but that's about it. I just can't count on him anymore. That really upsets me. I get lonely and tired. It doesn't seem fair. He's out having fun while I'm tied down with our baby. I never forced him to be a father. He was just as excited about parenting as I was. If it weren't for our daughter, I'd tell him to take a hike. That's how mad I get at him sometimes. I tell all my girlfriends to make their decision based on what they want to do and not what their boyfriends want them to do. I tell them if they think that they won't be able to handle being a mom without their boyfriend's support, then they should seriously look at their other options. I don't want to sound bitter, but you gotta know that you can't count on these guys. Think about his actions and not what he says he's going to do. My boyfriend has always done exactly what he's wanted to do. He's always thought of himself first. He's still doing that, only now he's got a baby.

Raising a child is hard work. Your boyfriend may not know what is expected of him as a parent and he may not be emotionally or financially ready to take on the responsibility. As was mentioned earlier, research has shown that teen dads more often come from disadvantaged backgrounds and have experienced difficulty in school. Becoming a parent places an additional financial and psychological stress on him when he's already experiencing other problems. Traditionally, the male role within a family has been viewed as the breadwinner. With today's economy, it may be difficult for your boyfriend to be successful in this role. It may be a blow to his self-esteem if he can't adequately provide for you and his baby.

Your boyfriend may not understand that his role as a father involves more than providing financial support. He may need help to understand the importance of his role. He may not have grown up with a father, and as a result may never have had a male role model. He may not have any positive role models to guide and support him. He may find it difficult to love and nurture his own child. It's very likely that he will also struggle with the changes in his lifestyle which will come with parenting. He may get tired of being a parent. The loss in his freedom and the changes in his social life may be too much for him. When he gets frustrated and finds parenting stressful, he may give up and leave the responsibility to you. It's important to establish clear boundaries with your boyfriend. Make sure you both know what you can expect from each other ahead of time. Be patient with your boyfriend as he learns his new role. You both can benefit from the support and guidance of an adult mentor or teen parenting program.

Teen dads are not all alike. It's a mistake to think that all teen dads abandon their parenting responsibility. Some teen dads are actively involved in raising their child. However, only a small minority of these dads will maintain long-term relationships with their children.

Keep in mind that parenting will be just as stressful for your boyfriend as it will be for you. Your boyfriend may experience conflict over wanting to be a good father and wanting to experience his adolescence without the burden of a child. Here's how Frank described his experience:

I was always trying to do the responsible thing. I got a part-time job after school. I stayed by my girlfriend's side through her entire pregnancy. Our baby was born early, and stayed in the hospital a long time. I got so frustrated trying to be at the hospital with my girlfriend and our son and trying to go to school and work. It was too much for me. Eventually I stopped going to school. It was the only way I could cope. I finally got some counseling for myself. I went back to school and learned how to deal with everything better. Our son is out of the hospital now. I take care of him a couple nights a week, and spend some time with him on the weekend. Now that I'm taking care of my own needs I'm enjoying parenting more. I love my son. I couldn't imagine not taking care of him and being there for him when he needed me.

If your boyfriend is willing, his participation should be encouraged. His involvement will benefit both you and your baby. His financial support will be a big help to you because early parenting has been associated with poverty for many teen moms. Your boyfriend's emotional support is also important. Having the father of your baby involved is likely to increase your sense of self-confidence and you may feel more secure knowing you can rely on him for support. Your boyfriend will also benefit from his involvement. He will feel more confident and will likely feel better about himself.

Most important, your child will benefit from his father's involvement. Research has shown that when fathers are voluntarily involved in the care of their children there is a positive effect. Fathers' participation has been shown to promote the child's cognitive development (the ability to learn and reason) and physical health as well as reduce the likelihood of behavioral problems in school.[9]

The father of your baby may not understand how vital his role is in your child's development. He may lack confidence in his ability to be a father. He may need your support and encouragement. Be patient with him as he takes on this new role which is probably unfamiliar to him. Fatherhood and motherhood are roles which are learned. It takes time to adjust to them. Typically, supportive services have been targeted for teen moms to help them adjust to pregnancy and parenting. In recent years support programs have been formed for teen dads to provide them the social services they need to help them develop as individuals and become better parents. Some teen dads express a desire to be better to their children than their own fathers, who were mostly absent while they were growing up. Some teen dads request counseling and voluntarily attend child development and parenting classes.

Some teen dads do not respond as eagerly to these support programs as do teen moms. Sometimes outreach strategies have ben needed by community workers to draw teen dads to these programs. Once teen dads know about these services and what they can expect, they usually respond positively. The services teen dads often request include child care and development classes, relationship counseling, and help with continuing their education and finding jobs. Teen dads who have stable relationships with the mothers of their children and who are already involved in their child's care are more likely to take part in these programs.

There aren't as many programs for teen dads as there are for teen moms, but these types of programs are growing as their services are becoming more popular. Your boyfriend can access a teen dad program operated in your community or run by the YMCA, or through existing programs that serve entire families. Your boyfriend is also welcome to come to your prenatal care appointments with you. Your prenatal care provider can oftentimes refer your boyfriend to a teen dad program, as well as refer you both to childbirth and parenting classes.

If your boyfriend does not feel comfortable attending a special program for teen dads, he may prefer to seek services from programs that serve all young males and not just fathers. These programs are usually associated with schools, churches, recreational programs, alcohol and drug detoxification programs, criminal justice programs, counseling programs, and employment and training programs. Only a few of these programs have specific services for fathers; however, they may offer other services which your boyfriend needs, such as life option programs and assistance with finishing school and finding a good job. Your boyfriend may need to take responsibility for his own personal growth before he can focus on parenting. These programs may offer the services he needs to take control of his life. He may also benefit from being with other men who are striving to better themselves and maintain healthy lifestyles.

The "Boys to Men" group is an example of a support group for young men held in an inner-city high school in Boston, Massachusetts. The support group meets once a week. All young men, including teen dads, are encouraged to attend. Mr. Sterling Anderson, a counselor in the area, runs the group and has this to say:

> Young men come to my group to talk about the fear, confusion, anger, frustration, and feelings of hopelessness that they have experienced. As a group, we help each other to identify personal feelings and other emotions and then relate them to the natural process of personal growth. I encourage

young men to accept responsibility for their own actions as part of taking care of themselves. I tell young men that if they have a child, then they are responsible for that child. I also remind them that they are responsible for their own personal growth and development. Dropping out of school to care for your child is not responsible. If you shut down your own personal development, your child's growth and development will also suffer. My motto is to be all that you can be.

One student who regularly attends the group explained why he participates: "Everyone is telling us what to do, but no one is showing us how to do it. The reason why we like coming to this group is because Mr. Anderson shows us how, and makes us feel we can accomplish anything we want."

Mr. Anderson encourages young men to learn more about themselves, to discover what they want out of life, to have personal goals, and to take the steps necessary to meet their goals. He encourages young men to get counseling whenever they're faced with the decision to become a teen parent. Early fatherhood can be stressful. Your boyfriend should reach out to positive role models, such as his father, uncle, teacher, or join a support group for young men, such as the one run by Mr. Anderson, or a program run by his church or other community group.

Establishing Paternity

No matter how your boyfriend feels about your pregnancy, he shares in the responsibility. Each state has laws regarding paternity (fatherhood), which a trained pregnancy counselor can explain to you. If you decide to raise your baby and you choose not to marry, establishing paternity is something you will need to think about. In other words, establishing paternity is the legal process of identifying the biological father of your baby. If you are not married, paternity needs to be established, preferably as soon as possible.

There are important benefits for you, your child, and your child's father to be gained from establishing legal paternity. Legal paternity must be established in order for your baby's father to have legal rights or legal responsibilities as a parent. It must be established before child support, visitation rights, or custody can be court ordered. If paternity has been established, children are also eligible for social security benefits and military benefits even if you are not married to the baby's father. Establishing paternity will provide your child with the legal documentation of who his father is, as well as give legal access to medical records. Your child may benefit emotionally from knowing who his father is. In some states now if the father's identity is not established your ability to receive public assistance payments may be jeopardized. You can begin the process of establishing legal paternity in the hospital after delivery of your child. If you have questions about this you should get legal advice as soon as possible.

Over one-third of teen moms do not identify the father of their baby. This is one of the major obstacles preventing collection of child support payments. If paternity was never established, a court cannot enforce child support even if the financial status of the father of your baby improves later in life. Establishing paternity can have emotional benefits for your baby's father. He can enjoy the emotional rewards that come from being a parent as well as having peace of mind that his child will be financially cared for if something should happen to him.

Things to Consider

- Early parenthood can have the same negative consequences for the father of your baby it has for you.
- Be open and honest with each other when deciding whether you will parent your child together. Parenthood is a long-term commitment, and it involves consequences to your child.
- Have realistic expectations of the emotional and financial support your boyfriend can provide.
- Allow your boyfriend, if he is willing, to participate in childbirth preparation, the birth of your child, and raising your child. Both you and your baby will benefit from his support.
- The father of your baby needs support and guidance for parenting as well as for dealing with issues in his own life. He will benefit from support programs.

Notes

1. National Center for Health Statistics, "Advance Report of Final Natality Statistics, 1990," *Monthly Vital Statistics Report* 41, no. 9 supp. (February 25, 1993), as cited in The Alan Guttmacher Institute, *Sex and America's Teenagers* (New York: Alan Guttmacher Institute, 1994), p. 53.

2. W. Marsiglio, "Adolescent Males' Orientation toward Paternity and Contraception," *Family Planning Perspectives* 25, no. 1 (1993): 22–31.

3. W. Marsiglio, "Adolescent Fathers in the United States: Their Initial Living Arrangements, Marital Experience and Educational Outcomes," *Family Planning Perspectives* 19, no. 6 (1987): 240–51, as cited in M. L. Sullivan, *The Male Role in Teenage Pregnancy and Parenting: New Directions for Public Policy* (New York: Vera Institute of Justice, Inc., 1990), p. 10.

4. Sullivan, *The Male Role.*

5. F. F. Furstenberg et al., *Adolescent Mothers in Later Life* (Cambridge: Cambridge University Press, 1987), as cited in Sullivan, *The Male Role.*

6. J. B. Hardy et al., "Fathers of Children Born to Young Urban Mothers," *Family Planning Perspectives* 21, no. 4 (1989): 159–63, 187.

7. K. A. Moore, *Facts at a Glance* (Washington, D.C.: Child Trends, 1987), as cited in J. J. Card and S. Nelson-Kilger, *Just the Facts: What Science Has Found Out about Teenage Sexuality and Pregnancy in the U.S.* (Los Altos, Calif.: Sociometrics Corp., 1994), p. 81.

8. Guttmacher Institute, *Sex and America's Teenagers,* p. 59.

9. Sullivan, *The Male Role,* p. 43.

11

Moving Forward

Everything in life has a beginning, a middle, and an end. Your life will not be the same as it was before your pregnancy. You will have grown because you will have suffered pain. There is personal growth and wisdom to be gained from this experience.

Hopefully by now you have begun to think through your options—adoption, abortion, and parenting—and you are working toward or have already made what you believe is the best choice for you. You should have talked to at least one adult you trust—a parent, teacher, health care provider, or counselor—in order to obtain as much information on each option as possible. No matter which choice you make, you will feel loss. This is normal. Share your feelings with the people you love and trust, and begin rebuilding your life. Remember to take precautions in the future so you do not put yourself in the position of having another unintended pregnancy. Talk to your health care provider about the various safe and reliable forms of contraception available, or speak to a counselor at a local clinic such as Planned Parenthood.

You may be finding this experience stressful. You are not alone. Over the years many young women have been faced with an unintended pregnancy. No doubt they felt, and perhaps were overwhelmed by, many of the same emotions that you have been experiencing: shock, denial, anger, guilt, and confusion. Many of these young women have shared their experiences, hoping that what they learned would help someone else. In the end, though, the decision is yours to make. No one can tell you what is right for you to do. You are the only one who knows the dreams you have for your life, and no one really knows how your future will be affected by what you do now.

Kerri's story is an example of how the future can unfold differently than expected. Her words may help you.

I was a teen mother. I turned eighteen on the day I graduated from high school and then, almost two weeks later, I found out I was pregnant. I was devastated and my parents thought it was the end of the world for everyone involved. The father of my baby moved two thousand miles away and, for a while, we kept in touch, but then we ended it. Eventually, we started to talk again. He was eighteen months younger than me and, even though I had already graduated from high school, he was a junior the year I was pregnant. We decided to get married that spring after he finished his junior year. He moved back to where we were from originally and he went to school for his senior year while I worked to support us. Then he joined the Air Force and we had our second child. We are now expecting our third and we have been married for four years. Getting married and continuing our life together was the best thing I have ever done. In a way, what seemed to be the worst possible scenario turned out to be a blessing. I wouldn't change anything. It has taken a lot of work and I had to go to school while I was pregnant so I could support myself and the baby after she was born. But the bottom line is that getting married and having a family when you're young is not always the end of things as you know them to be. Sometimes, it is just the beginning of a better life for everyone involved.

In the beginning my parents were not supportive at all and they hated the father. Now they love my kids more than life itself. They are more excited for our third than we are! I hope that this story can be an inspiration to teen moms because things aren't as bad as they seem. Things can work out in the end. You just have to be dedicated to finding the best route for yourself and don't let people tell you that you really messed up and ruined your life. Life is *not* over! And I hope I can be of some help to parents of teens who are pregnant, too. I hope they can see that there is hope for their daughters' and sons' lives that can be good and positive for everyone. Right now, parents need to be as supportive as possible and try to see that this is even harder for the kids than it is for them. Help the kids to make their own choices and try to love and support them no matter what decision they make. Good luck.

You may not make the same choice as Kerri, and that's okay. Not everyone is capable of being a good parent at a young age. But always remember: You have options.

Choice: Abortion

Choosing to terminate a pregnancy is often accompanied by feelings of guilt because it is necessary to admit to a mistake and to acknowledge that you are not willing to take responsibility for the child who would result from that mistake. Also, there are feelings of loss and wonder at what might have been in both your life and your child's life.

Once you have made the choice to have an abortion, you should be prepared for the emotional strain it may cause. Most people tend to feel guilt and sadness after an abortion; that is completely normal. You have lost part of yourself as well as part of your boyfriend. It may be harder to let that loss go if your boyfriend doesn't agree with your decision, and you may feel angry at his lack of support. You may question and regret your decision. Do not hold on to the pain and do not torture yourself with the feelings of regret. If you hold on to the pain and hurt all you will do is hinder your grieving process by taking energy away from more constructive parts of your life.

You might also, in the difficult process of this decision, lose the love of people around you. You might lose your boyfriend, but then just the idea of being a father—no matter what choice you might make—may make him turn and run. You might lose the love of people in your family who do not approve of your decision. The people who truly love you may not agree with your decision but will love you in spite of what has happened. You might lose respect among your extended family and the community. The clergy and the church to which you belong to may not agree with your actions, but no matter what, you will not lose the love of God.

You can expect that the decision you made may bring about a questioning of your religious and moral values. Be strong in knowing that you made what you believe was the best decision for yourself. If your boyfriend was not a part of your life and part of the decision, then having the abortion further removes a person from your life who would probably not be supportive of you in the future. It also allows you to see that person's "real" commitment and responsibility to you. If he does want to be part of your life once there is no baby to worry about anymore, you can make a good judgment of whether or not to resume your relationship. You must consider, however, that what happened this time is probably a good sign of what he will do the next time there is any problem.

Abortion carries with it a great emotional burden. However, in the end, it may require the least amount of adjustment in the way you live your life. You can continue in school as if nothing had happened, choosing when and with whom you share that part of your life. This may be the time for you to re-evaluate your own expectations of yourself as well as the type of relationships you want in the future. You may need to make some difficult decisions and change your behavior based on these evaluations. Perhaps a new group of friends with values which more closely match the way you now want to behave would be appropriate. Outward appearances may remain the same, but the changes within yourself can make you more committed to family, school, and work.

GRIEVING THIS LOSS

For those of you who are grieving after choosing abortion, we have the following advice and points for you to consider:

- Allow yourself to feel the pain. Allow yourself to grieve. The pain must be faced before you can move on.
- Give yourself time to grieve.
- Share your feelings with your friends, family, or boyfriend.
- Don't be afraid to seek professional help from a counselor or minister. They will help you. They will share your pain.
- If you have religious faith, talk to God. Remember, God forgives you and loves you.
- Forgive yourself. This is often the hardest part. But what's most important is that you cannot move on with your life without forgiving yourself.
- Avoid getting pregnant again. Take the necessary steps, either abstinence or the consistent, correct use of birth control, to prevent another unintended pregnancy.
- Reach out to other women who have had the same experience as you. Join or start a support group.
- Anniversaries may be painful for you. Spend them with a friend or relative. Share your burden.
- Don't be afraid to go on with your life. It is a great journey.

CHOICE: ADOPTION

If you have chosen adoption, like the other options, you will feel a sense of loss because you are giving up something that has been a part of you for nine months. You may feel sadness and loss because you will have no or limited contact with your child—the person you helped to create. The people around you may not agree with your decision and so you may feel a loss of their love and approval. You may have lost your boyfriend because he did not agree with your decision.

After making your adoption plan, you may find it difficult to face all those people, family and friends, who know of your pregnancy and your decision. The adoption agency with which you are working will be able to help you with these issues. Remember, without supportive people in your life the process of dealing with your feelings and of healing can be extra difficult.

The feelings you have are all understandable. You created a new life and nurtured it throughout your pregnancy. You can take pride and joy knowing that you are giving your child a better life than you could currently provide. You have also given a couple the opportunity to realize their dream of raising a child. The decision you made was a loving and selfless one.

Placing your child for adoption provides you with another chance to focus on your life's dreams without the responsibility for another human being who is totally dependent on you. Feel good about your decision. Enjoy your youth. Continue your education and pursue your life's dreams. Be comforted knowing that your child will be loved and cared for.

GRIEVING THIS LOSS

- Think about and focus on the valid reasons for making your decision.
- Realize that your child will be with parents who will be able to love and fully support him. You are giving your child a better life.
- You will grieve. Feel your loss. Talk to friends, a companion, and relatives who are supportive.
- Anniversaries may be painful for you. Spend them with a friend, a relative, or your boyfriend. Share your burden.
- Stay away from unsupportive and judgmental people. Be confident in the knowledge that your decision was the best for you and your baby.
- Realize that there will come a time when it is appropriate for you to have a child.
- Talk to God.
- Forgive yourself. Feel good about yourself and the decision you have made.
- Be positive about the future.

CHOICE: PARENTHOOD

This option requires the most effort from you right now and throughout your baby's life. There are more possibilities for both mistakes and successes. Your life will change from the day you decide to raise your child until the day you die. Motherhood means making sacrifices for your child.

You have chosen to accept a huge responsibility and you must plan how to best provide for both of your futures. Without education, the future may be limited, so you must try to continue in school. You may have to rely on your family or others to help you with expenses and support.

Your baby's father may be willing to take on his share of responsibility, but you cannot make assumptions based on promises from others. Statistics show that the older the children of single mothers get, the less contact they have with their fathers. Therefore, the responsibility of raising your child may rest wholly on your shoulders. Try to work to build whatever savings are possible. If your family is not supportive, remember there are groups and government programs that can help to provide food, housing, health care, and some of the support that you will need.

You may also need to take parenting classes and find a way to cope with growing up faster than you had planned. You must realize that your childhood is now over; it is now your baby's turn. In making this decision, you will give up many freedoms and good times to put the needs of your child first. You will no longer be able to come and go as you please. You will lose the independence that as a young adult you are just beginning to gain.

You will gain a little person who loves you, but you lose a lot of yourself in the process. You have to grow up and take responsibility. That means putting lots of attention, time, and money into your child's well-being. You must be responsible for doctor's visits, immunizations, and any other needs that your child has, whether it be in the middle of the afternoon or the middle of the night.

Having a baby who is dependent on you may make you feel needed and useful, which can boost your self-esteem; however, you may not feel quite as good about yourself if you find child rearing to be more than you expected. Your friends may or may not be a major part of you life as they were before. You will live a different life than most teenagers and your priorities will have to be different from theirs.

There is a possibility that your choice to parent will cause the loss of your relationship with your boyfriend. He may not be ready to assume the responsibilities of being a father, and your choice to raise your child could cause the relationship to end. You may also lose the love and approval of the family and friends around you. They may not agree with your choice and may withdraw their support.

One very unfortunate loss that many young pregnant teenagers face is the loss of some (if not all) of their hopes and dreams for the future (at least for the time being, if not forever). Hand in hand with that is the loss or the limiting of education. If education falls short of the minimum by today's standards—no high school diploma or GED and no other type of training such as technical, military, or post-secondary education—then you also lose the opportunity for higher paying jobs that would allow you to provide for your child in a better manner. A child also limits your job schedule flexibility and creates a need for outside help so you can work and support your child.

If you are willing to make these sacrifices they will be rewarded tenfold in the love and joy of raising a child. Teen parenting is a challenge, but it is *not* impossible. If you are truly committed to raising your child and are willing to make the necessary sacrifices, you will succeed. You will feel satisfaction and joy as you watch your child grow and thrive and discover the world around him. Being a good mother is a major accomplishment, one of which you should be proud.

TIPS FOR COPING WITH THE CHALLENGES OF PARENTING

- Recognize that motherhood is a full-time job.
- Begin planning now for your financial needs.
- Don't be afraid to ask for help. Participate in parenting classes or a support group.
- Maintain proper nutrition for you and your child. Ensure that you both receive adequate health care, including immunizations for your baby.
- Keep your education and personal goals in focus. Acknowledge that the plans you had made to achieve these goals may need to be altered somewhat now that you are going to be a mother.
- Determine who will be available and willing to help you with child care—your parents, another relative or friend, or perhaps your boyfriend.
- Surround yourself with people who share your values and goals and who will help and encourage you to reach these goals.
- Use effective contraception correctly and consistently to plan and space future pregnancies.
- Reward yourself occasionally. Do something nice for yourself, even if

it's only a relaxing bath while someone else watches the baby. Taking time for yourself will help give you the energy and enthusiasm you will need to cope with difficult times.

• Enjoy your child.

What about the Father?

Ethically and ideally all the men who are a part of unintended pregnancies would behave responsibly and be supportive of the mother's decision. That means he would not interfere with whatever choice she made.

If you choose to raise your child, whether or not you remain in a relationship, it is as much the father's responsibility as it is yours. The father's responsibilities include helping you through the pregnancy, being there for you and your child after the birth, and helping to raise his child. A father has a financial obligation, but most important for the child is the father's obligation to care for his baby. The father needs to devote time, attention, and love, as well as financial assistance. Unfortunately, many young men are not mentally and emotionally prepared to do this.

If the father of your child leaves after finding out you are pregnant, there are ways you can make him at least financially accountable through government laws and enforcement. This may take some time and money that you may not have, but there are people who are willing to help and a law that supports your efforts. In the long run it will make life easier for both you and your child.

If the father chooses to remain a part of the child's life but not yours, support his involvement. Don't deprive your child of a very important part of her life by denying her father contact.

Another choice for a your baby's father is to stick with you and help you raise your child on a daily basis. You may or may not be married, but he is committed to you and his child. He helps out with the child any time and is there to support you as well.

───

Pregnancy is a major event in any woman's life, and for a young, single woman, it can be very scary. The future may look bleak and dreary. You must always remember, though, *you have options*. The choice of how to handle this pregnancy is yours. You will need to gather information on all your choices and proceed in a calm and rational manner. Getting as many facts as possible about all your options will help you make the decision that you believe is best for you. Think back on all the information that has been presented to you in this book. Remember the stories of the young women who made the choice to parent their babies or place them for adoption, or who decided to have an abortion. Consult the resources, the clinics and public information groups, listed at the end of this book for answers to any questions you may still have. Be an active participant in the decision-making process. Take the necessary time to make a fully informed decision. Believe in yourself. Have faith in your ability to make the decision that is best for you.

And remember: Your life is not over because you are pregnant. It will change, but it will not end. Change is often painful, but you will survive, and you will be a stronger person as a result of your experience.

In life there are problems. Some have solutions. Some don't. Do not worry about things that you cannot change or affect. It saps your energy to be worried or anxious about a problem that you cannot change. Go on with your life.

For many years, we have worked with people in difficult situations, and through these experiences we have learned this important lesson: *Make today count.* The secret of life is learning to enjoy it. Go out and enjoy it. Enjoy the good days, the bad days, your dreams, disappointments, and successes; joy and anger, sorrow and happiness, hope and fear, indecision and strength. Allow your losses and grief to give you the ability to enjoy every day. Remember, the greatest tragedy of life is not that we are going to die, it is that we have not fully lived. Go out and live it. Adventure through your life.

Glossary

Abortion. The termination of a pregnancy before the fetus is capable of living outside the uterus. Abortions may be spontaneous, as in the case of a miscarriage, or they may be induced, that is, caused intentionally through medical intervention.

Adoption. The action of taking a minor who is not one's biological offspring into the legal relationship of a child.

Amniotic Sac. Also known as the bag of waters, this is the fluid-filled pocket in which the fetus develops. It is formed from membranes lining the uterine cavity.

Anemia. A deficiency of red blood cells or their hemoglobin sometimes due to a lack of iron in the blood. If you become anemic, you may be pale and tired.

Anesthesia. Medication used to numb the nerves. A *local anesthetic* will prevent feeling only in the area of the body on which the medical procedure is to be performed, while a *general anesthetic* will put you to sleep.

Birth Control. Methods of preventing pregnancy. Common forms include the pill, condoms, diaphragms, and various types of implants.

Blastocyst. The name for a fertilized egg in the earliest stages of pregnancy (that is, just after fertilization and implantation in the uterus). Later in the pregnancy it is called an embryo and then a fetus.

213

Cervix. A small opening at the neck of the uterus leading to the vagina. The cervix produces mucus which controls the flow of sperm into the uterus.

Cilia. Tiny hairlike structures that line the fallopian tubes. The cilia move the egg from the ovary to the uterus and the sperm in the reverse direction.

Conception. The moment at which the sperm and the egg join and a new life begins.

Condom. A sheath, usually made of rubber (latex), worn over the penis during sexual intercourse to prevent pregnancy or infection from a sexually transmitted disease.

Contraceptive. A device used in order to prevent a pregnancy from occurring. (See also **Birth Control**.)

Dilate. To make wider.

Dilation and Curettage (D&C). A medical procedure which is performed to empty the uterus. In this procedure the cervix is dilated and an instrument called a curette is used to scrape the walls of the uterus. This procedure is done in some abortions and after some miscarriages to remove the contents of the uterus.

Dilation and Evacuation (D&E). A medical procedure used for abortions performed up through the twenty-first week of pregnancy. Laminaria (sterile seaweed) is inserted into the cervical opening to dilate the cervix. The next day, the doctor injects the cervix with a local anesthetic and then uses dilators to widen it some more. The doctor then uses a vacuum suction machine and other instruments to remove the contents of the uterus.

Douche. A jet of solution directed into the vagina for cleansing purposes. Many people believe that douching is a form of contraception, but this is a myth. In fact, douching after sexual intercourse could push the sperm toward the uterus.

Due Date. The date on which a baby is expected to be born. This is calculated by determining the first day of your last period, subtracting three months, and then adding seven days.

Ectopic Pregnancy. A pregnancy in which the fertilized egg remains in the fallopian tube rather than implanting on the wall of the uterus. Ectopic pregnancies are dangerous to the mother and require immediate medical attention.

Egg. The female reproductive cell.

Ejaculate. To release sperm during male orgasm.

Embryo. The fertilized egg in a woman's uterus which will develop into a baby (if nothing occurs to interrupt the pregnancy). This term is used through the eighth week of pregnancy, after which it is called a fetus.

Fallopian Tube. The tube which carries the egg from the ovary to the uterus. Each woman has two fallopian tubes.

False Negative. A pregnancy test which has a negative result even though the woman is really pregnant.

Fetus. The name for a developing baby after the eighth week of pregnancy.

Gynecologist. A doctor who specializes in the care of women and their reproductive systems. (See also **Obstetrician,** as these medical specialties are commonly linked.)

Hemorrhage. An abnormal loss of blood. A hemorrhage is an emergency and requires immediate medical attention.

Hormone. A product of living cells that circulates in body fluids and has a specific effect on the activity of other cells. Commonly known hormones include estrogen, progesterone, and testosterone.

Human Chorionic Gonadotropin (HCG). A hormone produced during pregnancy. Pregnancy tests look for the presence of HCG to determine if a woman is pregnant.

Implantation. The process by which the fertilized egg (blastocyst) attaches itself to the uterine wall.

Induced Abortion. The term for an abortion brought about through medical intervention (as opposed to a miscarriage or spontaneous abortion), this term also describes a particular type of medical abortion performed late in the second trimester of pregnancy. This procedure must be done in a hospital. The doctor injects a solution through the abdomen and into the amniotic sac. Labor and delivery of the fetus then follow. This process is often followed by a D&C to insure that the uterus is completely empty.

Judicial Bypass. The process which allows a minor to obtain an abortion without parental consent in states which require such consent. To obtain a judicial bypass, you must appear before a judge and demonstrate that you are mature enough to make a decision without your parents' input.

Low-Birthweight. This term refers to babies born early who weigh less than five and a half pounds.

Menopause. The period in a woman's life when menstruation stops naturally. A woman who is past menopause no longer ovulates.

Menstrual Cycle. A series of changes which take place in a woman's body each month to prepare for pregnancy. First, the egg matures and is released from the ovary; then it travels through the fallopian tube; and, if conception occurs, it embeds itself on the uterine wall, where it develops during pregnancy. If conception does not take place, the egg dissolves and it and the uterine lining are shed during menstruation.

Menstruation. The final phase of the menstrual cycle, during which the uterine lining is shed because pregnancy has not occurred.

Midwife. An individual with experience or training in assisting women in labor and childbirth.

Minor. In almost every state for most purposes, a minor is defined as someone who is under the age of eighteen.

Miscarriage. Also known as spontaneous abortion, miscarriages are the unintentional ending of a pregnancy. They usually occur if there is something wrong with the developing baby.

Morning Sickness. Nausea, with or without vomiting, which occurs mainly in the first trimester of pregnancy due to changes in hormone levels.

Mutual Consent Registry. Adoption registries maintained in various states with which birth mothers and adult adoptees can list their names. By contacting a mutual consent registry both parties are letting it be known that they would like to arrange a meeting.

Obstetrician. A doctor who specializes in childbirth and the care of the mother before and after birth occurs. This medical specialty is often linked to gynecology.

Open Adoption. Although there is no formal definition, in general this is an adoption in which the biological mother takes an active role in the adoption process. She may have varying degrees of contact with the adoptive parents and possibly with the child. Although practices vary, in most open adoptions the birth mother has some kind of ongoing contact with the adopters and the child throughout the child's life.

Ovary. A small, almond-shaped gland which produces the egg and female hormones important to reproduction. Each woman has two ovaries, which lie just beneath the fallopian tubes, about four or five inches below the waist.

Ovulation. The release of a mature egg from the ovary. Ovulation occurs approximately once a month, alternating between the two ovaries, in women of childbearing age.

Parental Consent and Notification. Parents must usually give their permission for their minor children to receive medical treatment. Usually states allow teens to consent to their own health care in certain situations (such as treatment of sexually transmitted diseases, prenatal care, and family planning), but the laws vary from state to state. Your state may require that one or both of your parents be informed and/or consent before you can have an abortion if you are under eighteen. (See also **Judicial Bypass**.)

Penis. The male genital organ which contains the duct for the release of sperm.

Placenta. The organ which connects the fetus to the mother's uterus. The fetus is attached to the placenta by the umbilical cord. Oxygen and nutrients pass from the mother to the fetus through the placenta, which also protects the fetus by forming a barrier to block out some harmful substances.

Post-Partum Blues A feeling of sadness which often follows childbirth. These feelings are caused by a change in hormone levels as your body readjusts to no longer being pregnant.

Pregnancy Induced Hypertension (PIH). Also referred to as preeclampsia, this is a common medical complication to occur among pregnant teens. The disorder may be characterized by high blood pressure, swelling, and altered kidney function.

Pregnancy Test. A medical test which can be performed on either blood or urine samples which looks for the hormone HCG in order to determine if a woman is pregnant. Pregnancy tests may be done at home or in a lab, depending on the type of test being performed.

Prenatal Care. Medical attention and monitoring of the mother and fetus during pregnancy.

Preterm Labor. The onset of labor before thirty-seven weeks of pregnancy.

Progesterone. The female hormone that causes the uterus to undergo changes to provide a suitable environment for a fertilized egg.

Prostate Gland. The gland in men located at the base of the urethra which produces seminal fluid.

Quickening. The first fetal movements, which can be felt by the mother about five and a half months into the pregnancy.

Rhythm Method. A method of birth control in which pregnancy is prevented by avoiding sexual intercourse around the time when a woman is ovulating and therefore most fertile.

Scrotum. The pouch of skin in males which hangs below the penis and holds the testicles.

Semen. A sticky, whitish fluid produced in the male reproductive system that contains sperm, and is ejected during ejaculation.

Seminal Vesicle. Either of a pair of glands in men which secrete one of the components of semen.

Sexually Transmitted Disease (STD). Infections which are transmitted during sexual intercourse, such as gonorrhea, chlamydia, and AIDS.

Sperm. Male reproductive cells.

Sperm Ducts. Also known as the vas deferens, these are the ducts in men through which sperm travel from the testicles to the urethra.

Testicles. Male reproductive glands which produce sperm and the hormone testosterone. The testicles are located inside the scrotum.

Trimester. A period consisting of three months. Pregnancies in humans are divided into three trimesters, each of which lasts about twelve weeks.

Umbilical Cord. A cord containing blood vessels that connects the fetus to the placenta of its mother.

Urethra. A tube which carries urine from the bladder out of the body. In men, it also carries sperm out of the body.

Uterine Lining. The lining of the uterus which develops each month to prepare for a pregnancy. If pregnancy does not occur, this lining is shed during menstruation.

Uterine Perforation. A surgical complication in which the wall of the uterus is torn or perforated. This may result as a complication of an abortion and requires medical attention.

Uterus. A muscular, pear-shaped organ in which a baby develops during pregnancy.

Vacuum Aspiration. The most common method of first trimester abortions, this process also carries the least risk. After a general anesthetic is administered, the doctor dilates the cervix and then inserts a small, flexible tube into the uterus. A suction machine attached to the other end of the tube then draws out the contents of the uterus.

Vagina. A tubular passageway in women that connects the uterus to the outside of the body.

Vas Deferens. See **Sperm Ducts.**

WIC (Women, Infants, and Children). A federally subsidized program that provides coupons for nutritious, essential foods to women and children who qualify for such aid.

Womb. Another name for the uterus.

Zygote. The fertilized egg before it begins to divide which will develop into a baby.

Resources

Abortion: National Organizations/Referrals

REFERRALS

Check your local telephone directory in the Yellow Pages under "Abortion Providers," or call the following organizations for a referral:

Planned Parenthood Federation of America, Inc.
810 Seventh Avenue
New York, NY 10019
(212) 541–7800
(800) 230–PLAN

National Abortion Federation (NAF)
1436 U Street, NW
Suite 103
Washington, DC 20009
(202) 667–5881
(800) 772–9100
Monday through Friday, 9:30 A.M.–5:30 P.M. (EST)

An association of abortion providers and other parties who work in reproductive health and for abortion rights, NAF operates a toll-free hotline which provides referrals for abortion services and funding.

NATIONAL ORGANIZATIONS

Catholics for a Free Choice (CFFC)
1436 U Street, NW
Suite 301
Washington, DC 20009–3997
(202) 332–7995

This is a national educational organization that supports the right to legal reproductive health care, including family planning and abortion.

Religious Coalition for Reproductive Choice
1025 Vermont Avenue, NW
Suite 1130
Washington, DC 20005
(202) 628–7700

This is a national coalition representing Christian, Jewish, and other religious organizations who work together to preserve reproductive rights.

ALTERNATIVES TO ABORTION

Check your local telephone directory for the listings of the following organizations in your area:

Birth Right
Right to Life
Florence Crittenton Association

Also, many area churches, temples, etc., will be able to recommend organizations or services who can provide information and counseling on alternatives to abortion.

Adolescent Health Care Providers

Society for Adolescent Medicine
1940 East 40 Highway
Suite 120
Independence, MO 64055
(816) 224–8010

There are adolescent clinics and adolescent health care specialists practicing throughout the United States. Most adolescent clinics are affiliated with large teaching hospitals. If you would like a list of adolescent health care providers associated with the Society for Adolescent Medicine in your state, please send a self-addressed stamped envelope to Mrs. Edie Moore, at the above address.

Adoption: National Organizations

National Adoption Information Clearinghouse
5640 Nicholson Lane
Suite 300
Rockville, MD 20852
(301) 231–6512

This organization provides information on adoption, a list of birth parent/ adult adoptee search and support groups in your state, referrals to counselors who specialize in working with birth parents, and information on books and articles of interest to birth parents.

Center for Family Connections
2326 Massachusetts Avenue
Cambridge, MA 02140
in Massachusetts, call (617) 547–0909
in New York, call (212) 777–7270
in California, call (510) 287–8981

This is an educational and clinical resource center that helps individuals and families through the decision-making process associated with an unintended pregnancy. This is one of the few agencies in the United States to provide counseling and/or education on both pre- and postadoption issues. (This agency does *not* arrange adoptions.) By calling the Massachusetts phone number you may obtain referrals to individuals nationwide who are experts on adoption issues.

National Council for Adoption
1930 Seventeenth Street, NW
Washington, DC 20009
(202) 328–1200
Monday through Friday, 9:00 A.M.–5:30 P.M. (EST)

A national nonprofit organization that promotes adoption and is a continuing source of information for adoptive families and those seeking to adopt. In addition, this organization provides referral services for women with unplanned pregnancies.

The Adoption Center
391 Taylor Boulevard
Suite 100
Pleasant Hill, CA 94523
(800) 877–6736
Monday through Friday, 9:00 A.M.–5:00 P.M. (nationally)

This is a state-licensed adoption agency that specializes in open adoptions. This agency is able to work with clients nationwide.

Birth Control

Check your local telephone directory in the Yellow Pages under "Birth Control" or call Planned Parenthood for a referral:

Planned Parenthood Federation of America, Inc.
810 Seventh Avenue
New York, NY 10019
(212) 541–7800
(800) 230–PLAN

Please note: An adolescent clinic in your community can also provide you with help and information on contraception.

Birth Defects

March of Dimes
1275 Mamaroneck Avenue
White Plains, NY 10605
(914) 428–7100

Child Abuse

Child Help U.S.A.
Child Abuse Hotline
(800) 422–4453
24 hours a day, seven days a week

National Committee to Prevent Child Abuse
332 South Michigan Avenue
Suite 1600
Chicago, IL 60604
(312) 663–3520

This organization provides helpful written material on parenting, names and addresses of local chapters (which can detail your community's resources), and general information on child abuse and neglect.

Family Counseling/Crisis Counseling

INFORMATION

Family Service America's Public Service Information and Referral Line
11700 West Lake Park Drive
Milwaukee, WI 53324
(800) 221–2681
Monday through Friday, 9:00 A.M.–5:00 P.M. (CST)

This organization provides referrals to its member organizations for individual or family counseling, or support groups throughout the United States.

HOTLINES

National Runaway Switchboard
(800) 621–4000
24 hours a day, seven days a week

Please Note: There may be a wait to get through. This hotline provides crisis intervention and local referrals for teenagers, especially runaways, and their parents.

Nine Line
(800) 999–9999
24 hours a day, seven days a week

Please Note: There may be a wait to get through.

This extensive resource provides crisis intervention, counseling, referrals, and practical supports (for example, shelters, information and follow-up) to kids in trouble and to parents of runaways.

Prenatal Care, Childbirth, or Parenting Classes

Consult your school nurse or your health care provider who can help you find prenatal care and a comprehensive childbirth and parenting program for teens. You can also check your local telephone directory in the Yellow Pages under "Pregnancy."

Sexually Transmitted Diseases

HOTLINES

Centers for Disease Control HIV and AIDS Hotline
(800) 342–AIDS
24 hours a day, seven days a week

Spanish-language callers can dial
(800) 344–SIDA
8:00 A.M.–2:00 A.M. (EST), 7 days a week

Deaf callers needing TTY service can dial
(800) AIDS–TTY
Monday through Friday, 10:00 A.M.–10:00 P.M. (EST)

National Teen AIDS Hotline
(800) 440–8336
Friday and Saturday, 6:00 P.M.–Midnight (EST)

This hotline is staffed by trained teenagers who can talk to you about HIV and AIDS prevention.

Teens TAP (Teaching AIDS Prevention)
(800) 234–8336
Monday through Friday, 4:00 P.M.–8:00 P.M. (EST)

This hotline is staffed by teenagers who teach AIDS prevention.

Centers for Disease Control National Sexually Transmitted Disease Hotline
(800) 227–8922
Monday through Friday, 8:00 A.M.–11:00 P.M. (EST)

National Herpes Hotline
(919) 361–8488
Monday through Friday, 9:00 A.M.–7:00 P.M. (EST)

INFORMATION

American Social Health Association
P.O. Box 13827, Dept. AL
Research Triangle Park, NC 27709
(800) 230–6039
Monday through Friday, 9:00 A.M.–7:00 P.M. (EST)

Other Referral Services

Ask a Nurse
(800) 535–1111
Hours vary depending on where you live.

This organization refers callers to their local "Ask a Nurse" for questions on diseases and medical conditions. It also provides referrals to local doctors and community services.

Depression after Delivery Information Request Line
P.O. Box 1282
Morrisville, PA 19067
(800) 944–4PPD

This organization provides educational materials and referrals for women
and families coping with mental health issues associated with childbearing,
both during and after pregnancy.